PRAISE FOR
Quality Care, Affordable Care

"A seminal resource at a critical time! Dr. Shapiro unveils the complex relationships between stakeholders in the changing healthcare environment in America, demystifying the thought processes and motivations of doctors, insurers and patients, alike. ⌐ ⌐ ⌐ ⌐ examples from his team's work, Dr. Shapiro ou   ct maximum value (quality/cost), deta   n-led, data-driven standard development,   nally appropriate care of the highest qua

ERICA WEIRICH, MD
Director, Global Health Research Foundation
Adjunct Clinical Assistant Professor of Medicine
Stanford University School of Medicine

"In his new book, *Quality Care, Affordable Care*, Dr. Shapiro provides a novel solution to bending the cost curve and improving patient outcomes, a physician's perspective and recipe for success in an increasingly value conscious health care market. The book provides much needed fresh insight that takes the mystery out of medical cost reduction through a practical program of variation reduction—and puts the solution back in the hands of physicians.

As an experienced physician and health care administrator, Shapiro provides his proven formula for eliminating unnecessary, costly and potentially risky medical care while providing greater value to the patient through improved outcomes."

KARL G. SYLVESTER, MD
Associate Professor of Surgery and Pediatrics
Executive Director, Center for Fetal and Maternal Health
Lucile Packard Children's Hospital
Stanford University School of Medicine

"Formal guidelines are applicable to only a small fraction of clinical practice. Dr. Shapiro engagingly shows how groups of physicians asking questions about variations in their own practices can develop, and then adhere to, their own guidelines. Creating such learning healthcare systems is the best way to increase value in health care."

HAROLD S. LUFT, PHD
Caldwell B. Esselstyn Professor Emeritus of Health Policy and Health Economics
University of California, San Francisco
Author, *Total Cure: the Antidote to the Healthcare Crisis*

Quality Care, Affordable Care

HOW PHYSICIANS CAN REDUCE VARIATION

and

LOWER HEALTHCARE COSTS

LAWRENCE SHAPIRO, MD

GREENBRANCH
PUBLISHING

Phoenix, Maryland

13   8 7 6 5 4 3 2 1

Copyedited, typeset, indexed, and printed in the United States of America

CPT™® is a registered trademark of the American Medical Association

PUBLISHER
Nancy Collins

EDITORIAL ASSISTANT
Jennifer Weiss

BOOK DESIGNER
Laura Carter
Carter Publishing Studio

INDEX
Robert Saigh

COPYEDITOR
Pat George

To my wife, Maryellen,

Without your love, patience, and reassurance

I could not have written this book.

And to my grandchildren, Ellie, Samantha, and Colin,

whose need for a value-driven healthcare system

motivates me to do this work.

Table of Contents

Acknowledgments

Numerous people have contributed both to the development of the variation-reduction program at PAMF and to this book. I would like to thank Dr. Richard Slavin for giving me the time to develop the systems we would eventually use to create the variation-reduction project, Dr. Laurel Trujillo, who changed the focus of variation reduction from reducing cost to increasing value, and Dr. Wendi Knapp for transforming the project into an ongoing program by developing a methodology to train new variation-reduction champions. Without these three individuals, I do not believe this process or this book would have been possible.

I would also like to thank the other variation-reduction team members, whose hard work and steadfastness in the method have made this program successful: Dr. Jimmy Hu, Dr. Sue Knox, Dr. Veko Vahamaki, Dr. Laura Holmes, Serwar Ahmed, Lydia Paul-Flores, Betsy Stone, Ana Diaz, Tamara Smith-Jones, and Tiffany Bailey. Together, you continue to be the most functional team I have ever had the honor to work with.

Thank you to Lynn Segal, who first introduced me to the idea of the one-down approach and who made me realize that while data was necessary, the discussion was more important. Your counsel and friendship have kept me on course despite the turbulent times in healthcare.

Thank you to Beth Macom, a great editor and tireless taskmaster, for guiding me through the process of creating a book.

Thank you to Nancy Collins and the staff of Greenbranch Publishing for supporting me in this project and all the help in mentoring me through the maze of publishing a book.

Thank you to Dr. Melissa Welch, the Aetna Medical Director, who not only put up with all my phone calls and complaints about the Aetna data set, but led me to the realization that I needed to develop a data set of our own.

Thank you to the Information Technology Department of PAMF, without whose ongoing support this project could not have gotten off the ground, let alone taken off. In particular, I would like to thank Jocelyn Chan, who set up the initial data warehouse, and Pragati Kenkare and Cliff Olson, who maintained it just for me long after everyone else had migrated to a different system.

Thank you to Eric Nguyen, who is one of the smartest data analysts I have ever worked with, and who has taken our data management from cottage industry to industrial-strength process.

Thank you to Vicki Amon-Higa and Cyndee Bockinger-Lake, experts in lean organizations, who helped us move variation reduction from a pilot project to the way we practice medicine at PAMF.

Thank you to Dr. Neil Baker for giving me the opportunity to work with IHI on their white paper on appropriate use of specialty care, and for the many hours of discussion on how we can spread this type of work.

Thank you to Dr. Michael van Duren for helping to spread variation reduction to the rest of the Sutter Health system.

Thank you to the many physicians from 25 different departments at PAMF who have participated in variation-reduction meetings. Without your willingness to come to the meetings, respond to the data, and discuss how you care for patients, variation reduction would not have been possible.

Thank you to my parents, Herman and Dorothy Shapiro, who not only started me on my path in medicine but also showed me through their experiences in managing a family business how important it is to provide value to the customer.

And lastly, but most importantly: to my wife, Maryellen, my most honest critic, my strongest support, and my best friend, thank you.

About the Author

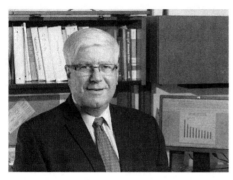 Lawrence Shapiro, MD, is a board-certified pulmonologist who throughout his career has been actively involved with the issues of appropriateness and utilization. His first practical experience in this area was as the chair of his hospital's intensive care unit, where he was faced with the issue of utilization of scarce resources. Later he became the utilization review medical director for the hospital. When he left solo practice for group practice he was asked to lead the group's managed care efforts. Since 2005 he has been the managed care medical director for the Palo Alto Medical Foundation, a large multi-specialty medical group in Northern California consisting of more than 1200 physicians in 30 locations in the San Francisco Bay area.

He has been involved with California's Integrated Healthcare Association's pay for performance as a steering committee member. On a national basis he has been on the faculty for the Institute for Healthcare's prototypical community on Appropriate Use of Specialty Care.

He was born in Brooklyn, New York, raised on Long Island, and moved to California to attend UCLA as an undergraduate. He graduated UCLA *magna cum laude* with a B.A. in psychology and was accepted to medical school at the University of California, San Francisco. He completed his medical degree in 1974 and returned to New York for his internal medicine residency at Kings County Hospital–Downstate Medical Center. In his final year of residency he was the chief resident in Internal Medicine. Realizing that California was the place to be, he returned to Harbor–UCLA Medical Center for his pulmonary fellowship where he was awarded an American Lung Association Training Fellowship.

He has been an invited speaker on the topic of affordability through variation reduction at numerous national and regional meetings, including the

Institute for Healthcare Improvement National Forum, the Integrated Healthcare Association, the Group Practice Improvement Network, and the California Association of Physician Groups.

He lives in Cupertino, California, with his wife of 41 years, Maryellen. They have two children and three grandchildren.

For the latest information on variation reduction please visit www.variation reduction.net

Introduction

This morning as I drove to work at the Palo Alto Medical Foundation, I listened to President Barack Obama deliver his second inaugural address. Just seven minutes into his speech, the president said, "We, the people, still believe that every citizen deserves a basic measure of security and dignity. We must make the hard choices to reduce the cost of healthcare and the size of our deficit."

This was the second of what would turn out to be the speech's five "We, the people" declarations, and I found it particularly satisfying not only that the president mentioned healthcare cost so prominently in this important speech, but also that he clearly linked its reduction to the major economic issue facing the country: reduction of the federal deficit. In these few words, President Obama transcended the controversy of the previous four years—healthcare *reform*—to address the core of the issue: healthcare *cost*. How "We, the people" should accomplish this task while preserving and even enhancing the quality of American healthcare is the subject of this book.

◆ ◆ ◆

When the president first proposed the ideas that would become the Affordable Care Act (ACA), many physicians in leadership positions took a wait-and-see attitude towards the looming changes in healthcare. Before we took actions of our own, some of us wanted to wait and see if the ACA would pass. Some of us wanted to wait and see if the Supreme Court would uphold it. Some of us wanted to wait and see if the 2012 presidential election would protect it. Now that those issues are settled, some of us still want to wait—this time to find out how many of our patients will be insured under ACA or how the insurance exchanges set up by ACA will reimburse us or how the proposed Accountable Care Organizations (ACOs) will work. But the change that President Obama promised more than four years ago is here, now, and it's time for us to act.

Certain provisions of the Affordable Care Act have already taken effect, such as allowing children to remain on their parents' health insurance until age 26 and removing restrictions on pre-existing conditions in children. In 2014, the individual-mandate provision will take effect, adding millions of Americans to the rolls of those with health insurance. Full implementation of the ACA is expected to improve healthcare in the United States by allowing people to obtain necessary care without fear of the financial burden they would face if required to pay for all care out of their own pockets. That financial burden is growing at an alarming pace: in 1980, the United States spent 10% of our gross domestic product (GDP) on healthcare. By 2000, the percentage was 14%. Currently, it's about 18%.[1] Most other industrialized countries in the world achieve similar quality as the United States, but spend much less on healthcare.[2]

The Act itself is a massive document, thousands of pages long. Some of its measures, such as funding for innovation, may eventually decrease healthcare expenditures, but overall, the Affordable Care Act is not healthcare reform; it's health *insurance* reform. Like Medicare, the ACA stipulates who will pay for care, not how much that care will cost, let alone set standards for its quality. The ACA itself will not arrest the increasing cost of healthcare in the United States.

Affordability and quality of healthcare are a keen interest of the Palo Alto Medical Foundation (PAMF), where I am a board-certified pulmonologist and have been the Managed Care Medical Director since 1998. PAMF was founded more than 75 years ago; for the past 40 years, the foundation has been heavily involved with improving quality of care and controlling the costs of healthcare through our HMO plans. Twenty-five years ago, PAMF became a community-based, not-for-profit medical foundation. As such, it has three functions: to provide healthcare for our community, to provide health education, and to promote healthcare-related research.

Since 2009, when PAMF fully implemented the innovative program that's the subject of this book, physicians at PAMF have reduced the cost of healthcare to our patients by more than $10 million per year while maintaining our "top performing group" status in the statewide, publicly reported quality measures sponsored by the Integrated Healthcare Association, the organization that sponsors the pay-for-performance program and monitors quality of healthcare in California. When I give presentations to medical industry audiences on how we've achieved these remarkable results, one of the first slides I show is a picture of my two beautiful granddaughters. I do this to underscore the reason I'm involved with the struggle to decrease total healthcare expenditures: according to the Congressional Budget Office (CBO), healthcare amounts to $1.38 trillion annually, which is 28% of the federal budget.[3] Without substantial changes, the federal debt will increase to 70% to 90% of GDP by 2022. Together, healthcare and social security are projected to increase by 62% in the next 10 years; the vast majority of that increase is healthcare-related.[4] Unless we curb its rising cost, healthcare will consume the resources of the United States to such an extent that we will not be able to provide the schools, roads, parks, libraries, and other public goods that my granddaughters and their peers will need in the coming years.

On the day that the Supreme Court upheld the ACA, President Obama said that the decision was a victory for all Americans. He related the story of a woman who had survived a cancer for 10 years, but each year her insurance company raised her rates to the point where she could no longer afford to keep her insurance coverage, and she was left to rely on chance alone to preserve her health. While the ACA may help that woman and allow her to purchase affordable health insurance, I don't believe that it will help my granddaughters' need for a healthy society in which to live. As citizens, we should not have to choose between the two; as physicians, we have an affirmative responsibility not only to our individual patients, but also to the community at large. As President Obama said, we Americans need to make the hard choices on both healthcare cost reduction and reducing the federal deficit. And we physicians are the ones who should lead in this effort.

Is there a true conflict between the individual and the community with regard to healthcare? Some would say that it should be patients' choice to decide what healthcare they should receive, even if that healthcare is not medically necessary. In an unbounded market, that might be true, but because only a finite amount of healthcare is available, the community needs to make choices to ensure that basic adequate care is available and affordable for all. A way to honor both the individual and the community is to make sure that the care that's provided is *valuable*—that is, that it's appropriate, of high quality, and cost-efficient.

◆ ◆ ◆

This book is the result of a program that PAMF began in 2005 to increase value in healthcare. With the support of then–regional President Richard Slavin, MD, who later became the foundation's CEO, I had the good fortune to lead several pilot projects to engage my colleagues in reducing common clinical practices that lead to unwarranted variation in healthcare. Using data from our billing systems, my project team was able to share unblinded data with physicians at PAMF showing how their individual and group practice patterns affected both cost and quality of care. The results of our limited pilot projects were so promising that we gained permission to implement the program throughout the foundation in 2009. By the end of 2012, physicians at PAMF had created standards that benefitted more than 130,000 patients and saved more than $31.3 million.

This book is written for physicians, physician leaders, and administrators of physician groups who want to take action to improve healthcare while reducing its cost. My goal for the book is to convince you that increasing value in the healthcare you provide is crucial to both your patients and the community and that variation reduction offers you the tools to accomplish that goal.

Part I of this book details the path that PAMF took toward variation reduction and the results we obtained. Part II discusses the reasons for undertaking such a program and the changes in thought and practice necessary to implement it. Part III is a "cookbook" with tips for how you can become master chefs by creating your organization's own local version of variation reduction.

Neither the program nor this book would have been possible without the specialists who worked on these projects, especially the variation-reduction physician champions. In particular, I'd like to thank Laurel Trujillo, MD, PAMF medical director for quality, and Wendi Knapp, MD, PAMF associate medical director for variation reduction, my partners on the PAMF variation-reduction steering committee.

Part I:

The Path to Variation Reduction

CHAPTER 1

Unwarranted Variation

I n 1967, Jack Wennberg, then a young physician working in Vermont under a Medicare-sponsored grant, noticed distinct geographic variations in surgical procedures performed in the hospitals of New England. The rates of operations at one hospital versus another appeared to be medically unnecessary; that is, they seemed to have more to do with how many surgeons were at a particular hospital, and where they had trained, than whether a particular area had a higher incidence of an illness or condition. Dr. Wennberg called this phenomenon "unwarranted variation"—healthcare whose delivery could not be explained by illness, medical need, or the dictates of evidence-based medicine.

In one small town in Vermont, for example, surgeons had removed the tonsils of 70% of children 15 and under; in another town just two hours away, the percentage was only 7%.[5] Intuitively feeling that 70% of children did not have diseased tonsils, Wennberg reviewed the data with the physicians who were removing tonsils at that elevated rate. They were surprised to learn of their collective overutilization.[6] When Wennberg asked them to begin seeking second opinions on the need for tonsillectomies, they agreed, and over a five-year period, their common attention to the issue enabled them to reduce tonsillectomy rates by two-thirds, eliminating unnecessary medical procedures and creating significant cost savings for patients.

PREFERENCE VERSUS SUPPLY

As he continued his research, Wennberg began to examine Medicare expenditures for other types of procedures. (Because Medicare has kept records since its inception in 1965, it's an invaluable source of data for researchers who want to understand the how, how much, and to whom of healthcare in the United States.) He found that he could classify Medicare expenditures into three categories:

1. What he called effective care, grounded in evidence-based medicine, comprised only about 12% of all Medicare expenditures.
2. Preference-sensitive care, driven mainly by the patient's desire to obtain a certain test or procedure, amounted to 25% of Medicare expenditures.
3. Supply-sensitive care, delivered at the discretion of the physician, accounted for 63% of all Medicare expenditures. This largest bucket of care was based not on medical evidence, but on expert opinion, and because experts' opinions vary, physicians could find an expert opinion to justify their varying decisions to test, prescribe, or operate.

When Wennberg found unwarranted variation in the small amount of evidence-based care, it was generally in the form of under-utilization of procedures; that is, physicians did less than they should have in caring for their patients. (And when unwarranted variation occurs as under-utilization, the cost is often measured in lives, not money. A recent example of under-utilization is physicians' failure to use beta blockers after an acute myocardial infarction. While the evidence is clear in the literature that using beta blockers saves lives, the utilization nationwide of this life-saving regimen is only about 60%.[7])

But in the large majority of cases (preference-sensitive and supply-sensitive care), the pattern of variation was towards over-utilization. Because this book concerns those two latter categories, my focus is on over-utilization of medical procedures.

Wennberg submitted his findings to the prominent medical journals of the day, but encountered multiple obstacles to publication: most editors could not believe that individual physician practices could vary so much just on the basis of personal preference of physicians. When his work was finally published in 1973, it appeared in *Science*, a journal that typically publishes basic research, not clinical studies, and was barely noticed by the medical community.[8]

WARRANTED VERSUS UNWARRANTED

Indeed, it remains difficult today for many physicians to believe in unwarranted clinical variation, even when shown the data. It's all too easy to think of other, more palatable, *warranted* reasons for variation in patient care, such as:

- The data are wrong.
- The data are correct but anomalous.
- My patients are sicker than other groups of patients.
- My medical group provides better service.
- We use different codes for that procedure or diagnosis.

And, in fact, some variation in treatment *is* warranted. Some physicians take care of patients with higher levels of acuity; or they are referred more patients for procedures because of an ability to perform a particular procedure that no one else in the area has the capability to do; or the population the physicians serve is truly different from the norm because of ethnic or socioeconomic characteristics. But unwarranted variation occurred in 1967 and it occurs through the present day.

While problems with unwarranted variation have been identified for nearly 50 years, little systematic success has been achieved in reducing that variation. Part of the problem may be that when discussing this issue there's no standard term used in either the medical or popular literature. The Institute for Medicine calls this issue "waste" and the Institute for Healthcare Improvement (IHI) calls it "overuse."[9] The National Quality Forum speaks of "misuse,"[10] while noted health economist Victor Fuchs calls it "not cost-effective."[11] Opponents to change speak of "rationing" and "death panels."[12] These later characterizations are not inventions of Sarah Palin and her ilk. As a teenager in the fall of 1962, I recall reading a *Life* magazine article on a "life and death committee" for allotting dialysis slots. As a medical student in the early 1970s, I remember discussing which of our patients would go on chronic dialysis, because even at that time a limited number of dialysis machines were available. Physicians have always agonized over these decisions, weighing the risks and benefits of every procedure and prescription. Politicizing the decisions does not make our choices any easier. Yes: sometimes our decisions are a matter of life and death, but that's part of what physicians do.

◆ ◆ ◆

VALUE

The difference between variation that's warranted and variation that's unwarranted is a difference in *value*. Traditionally, value in healthcare treatment is defined as the quality of the service (which is made up of clinical outcomes, ready availability of the service, and patient satisfaction) divided by the cost of the service:[13]

$$Value = \frac{Outcomes + Access + Satisfaction}{Cost\ to\ Patient}$$

or, more simply,

$$Value = \frac{Quality\ of\ Care}{Cost\ to\ Patient}$$

But, as Wennberg's work shows, there's an additional factor that's impact is enormous: the appropriateness of the procedure.[14] A physician can perform the highest-quality procedure at the lowest cost, for example, but if it's the wrong procedure, or done on the wrong patient, its value is negative. Consider the high rate of removal of tonsils in some Vermont children. Everything in a given surgery may have gone flawlessly and quickly, the surgery may have been scheduled for the time and in the location the parents wanted, and the parents may have been highly satisfied with the surgeon, hospital, and outcome, but if the child's tonsils didn't really need to be removed, the overall outcome was poor. So the value equation actually looks like this:

$$Value = \frac{Appropriateness \times Quality}{Cost\ to\ Patient}$$

Value must be the focus and the measure for improvement in healthcare. It doesn't matter if we're talking about improvement in clinical outcomes or improvement in how much we spend, value must be our main concern. Reducing cost without considering its effect on quality of care is folly, while a change that increases cost but also increases quality is something we intuitively know is valuable. The question is: how can we afford to make these improvements when the cost of healthcare is already so high?

AFFORDING THE NEW

I suggest that the only way we'll be able to afford the new and improved is to eliminate the inappropriate and unnecessary. I am not suggesting that new is always better than old. On the contrary, some older medications, tests, and procedures are still extremely useful. Aspirin has been around for more than 100 years and is still an effective and inexpensive anti-inflammatory medication, yet many doctors prescribe brand-name non-steroidal anti-inflammatory agents when generic aspirin will do. A simple test such as a chest X-ray can still diagnose many pulmonary problems, yet many physicians order the more costly and higher radiation of a CT scan even before obtaining the plain chest X-ray. Traditional surgery under local anesthesia is still an effective way to repair inguinal hernias, yet some surgeons now repair them through a laproscope, which requires general anesthesia. Many hospitals are adding robotic surgery units in an arms-race type competition with neighboring hospitals, even though there is little evidence that robotic surgery improves outcomes or decreases complications.

So before we choose to substitute new for old, we need to be clear that the change brings a gain in value. Does the benefit to this patient significantly outweigh the risk? If it does, then the value of the medication, test, or surgery is warranted; that is, it's high enough to make it a necessary and appropriate part of this patient's healthcare. *Warranted*, *necessary*, and *appropriate* are the keys to providing the care we all want, at a cost that we all can afford.

◆ ◆ ◆

THE DARTMOUTH ATLAS

After leaving Vermont, Jack Wennberg joined the faculty of Dartmouth School of Medicine, where he founded the Center for Evaluative Clinical Sciences and expanded his research into variation to the national level. One of his achievements is the Dartmouth Atlas of Health Care (www.dartmouthatlas.org), a series of colorful maps of the United States that use increasingly saturated hues to display low-, medium-, and high-utilizing areas of various Medicare services. Whether the data represented are for hospital use, surgical procedures, post-acute care, or any other of a number of topics, map after map shows the same vast, unwarranted geographical variations in care.

One of the most intriguing of the Dartmouth Atlas maps (see Figure 1) shows Medicare expenditures in the last six months of life. This map shows the same kind of geographic variations that all the others do and is quite convincing even to those who are skeptical about the reality of unwarranted

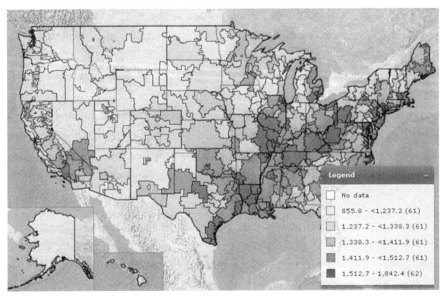

Legend

☐ No data
☐ 855.8 - <1,237.2 (61)
☐ 1,237.2 - <1,338.3 (61)
☐ 1,338.3 - <1,411.9 (61)
▨ 1,411.9 - <1,512.7 (61)
■ 1,512.7 - 1,842.4 (62)

FIGURE 1. Medicare expenditures in the final months of life (in dollars). Used by permission from the Dartmouth Atlas of Health Care.

variation in healthcare: because these patients all had the same outcome (they died), it would be hard to insist that costs were higher in some areas because some patients were sicker than others.

McALLEN, TEXAS

One of the hot spots on Dartmouth Atlas maps is the city of McAllen, at the southern tip of Texas. In 2006, McAllen had one of the highest per-capita expenditures for Medicare in the United States; Medicare spent $15,000 per enrollee there, almost twice the national average and more than twice that of El Paso, another Texas border town with similar demographics. Unfortunately, the quality of that care as measured by Medicare was no better than average; in some McAllen hospitals, it was below average. Why the inflated expense?

Atul Gawande, a Harvard-based surgeon, MacArthur Fellow, and staff writer for *The New Yorker*, interviewed numerous physicians in the McAllen area. He also spoke with experts at Dartmouth's Institute for Health Policy and Clinical Practice and examined information from companies such as Ingenix, a data-analysis company owned by UnitedHealthcare. The answer he got from all these sources was the same: physicians in McAllen ordered more diagnostic testing, performed more surgery, recommended more hospitalizations, and, in general, prescribed more of everything.[15] In McAllen, which Dr. Gawande called "a system with no brakes," as in some of the small towns of Vermont, individual decisions of physicians resulted in clinical variation that compounded into systematic over-utilization and skyrocketing costs.

This time, the account of conspicuous unwarranted variation did not go unnoticed; Gawande's *New Yorker* article about over-utilization in McAllen garnered national attention. And at the December 2009 National Forum of the Institute for Healthcare Improvement (IHI)—one of the most influential forces for improvement in care in both the United States and the world— White House staffers involved with creating healthcare reform legislation mentioned that President Obama had made the article required reading for all staffers, not just those working on the healthcare issue.

For now, McAllen, Texas, may be an outlier, but as long as the U.S. healthcare system continues to reward doctors for doing *more* rather than for doing *what's appropriate*, it will be difficult to attain the goal of affordable healthcare for all Americans.

We in the medical profession have an obligation to the healthcare system to pull "appropriateness" into our thinking about value to reduce unwarranted variation in treatment—not only the wild, blatant (and we hope isolated) variation exemplified by McAllen, but the quiet, pervasive variation caused by the current way that most physicians and medical groups practice medicine.

ISN'T THIS RATIONING?

This book is not about rationing care. It's about doing the right thing for the right patient. To those who want to rant about rationing, I say that healthcare is already rationed today. Unfortunately, it's not an ethical rationing of care—one that provides services to those who need them— it's an economic rationing that provides services to those who can afford them. The Institute of Medicine estimates that fully 30% of healthcare in the United States is inappropriate and offers no value to the patient.[16] If we eliminate this unnecessary care, our healthcare system will have the ability to provide—and pay for—what is truly of value to the patient.

So how do we get to appropriately valued care? We know what doesn't work: we experienced it in the managed care era of the 1990s, when HMOs sprang up like mushrooms after rain. Every one of these organizations had administrators who produced volumes of clinical guidelines that physicians were to follow or care would be denied. This top-down approach grated on both physicians and patients. Physicians felt that they had no say in how they were to treat their patients. Patients felt that a nameless, faceless HMO medical director who had never seen them was preventing them from getting the care they needed. And both were right: it became obvious to both the physicians and the patients that the goal of the for-profit, publicly traded HMOs was to increase profits by reducing patient care. So while it's true that fee-for-service medicine has an inherent incentive to do more, which is problematic, just as bad was the HMO incentive to reduce cost at the expense of the patient. Neither approach works; we need to do something entirely different.

SOMETHING DIFFERENT

That something is variation reduction, as initiated and practiced by physicians. If we're serious about the goal of affordable healthcare for all Americans, we physicians need to lead the way. Most healthcare in the United States is ordered or directed by physicians. We order the tests, prescribe the medication, and do the surgery. These are the activities that increase the cost of care in the United States each year. In the absence of robust evidence-based medicine, physicians must command the tools to determine what the standard of care should be and possess the autonomy to enact it.

Variation reduction is a system that engages physicians by making transparent the differences in our practices. It encourages physicians to discuss our different practice styles and come to an agreement on what is standard work for a particular clinical problem. Variation reduction is a bottom-up, physician-centric tool to encourage physicians to work together to create local standards of care and engage us to provide consistent, appropriate care even where there is no evidence-based medicine.

The data in Jack Wennberg's Dartmouth Atlas shows variation among regions. It even shows variation among individual hospitals within regions. What it doesn't show is variation among physicians. What if you could analyze and reduce variation on the level of individual physicians? While the concept of clinical variation is not new, what is new is how we can use our understanding of variation as an instrument for change.

◆ ◆ ◆

This first chapter introduced the concept of variation reduction and argued for the need to incorporate "appropriateness" into our traditional definition of "value." The remaining chapters of Part I trace the path that PAMF took to arrive at variation reduction. In Chapter 2, I discuss a failed national attempt to define and enforce ideas about "appropriate use" and PAMF's own first successes. Chapter 3 follows a major health plan's unsuccessful attempts to tier PAMF physicians based on "efficiency," and the lessons we learned from the attempt. Chapter 4 introduces PAMF's initial steps in variation reduction, from pilot project to full implementation. Chapter 5 details the success of our results.

CHAPTER 2

Inappropriate Use

A t the 2009 meeting of the Institute for Healthcare Improvement, outgoing IHI president and CEO Donald Berwick delivered a challenging speech, one of his last before beginning his abbreviated term as head of the U.S. Centers for Medicare & Medicaid Services. (Because Berwick was so outspoken on healthcare issues, he ran afoul of D.C. politics and was never confirmed by the Senate. After serving a 16-month term via a presidential recess appointment, he left to become a fellow of the Center for American Progress.)

Berwick and colleagues founded IHI in 1991 to apply systems thinking to meet important social needs in healthcare. Its triple aim was to foster better care, better health, at lower cost.[17] In his keynote speech, Berwick chided attendees that while the organization had long prided itself in both improving quality of care and improving the health of populations, it had done little to improve affordability; if IHI as an organization was going to fulfill its mission, it had to take on this last and difficult part of the triple aim.[18]

IHI'S FRAMEWORK

In response to Berwick's challenge, IHI leadership reviewed the literature on the cost of U.S. healthcare and found that care ordered by specialists was a significant source of unnecessary spending. Reducing unnecessary specialty care would free the dollars that were going for unnecessary care to support the goal of universal coverage. It would also help keep quality high and decrease risk to the patient. In 2010, IHI published a white paper on cost reduction through "appropriate use" of specialty services.[19] The paper offered a six-step framework that organizations could use to develop their own programs to reduce unnecessary care:

1. Engage physicians, patients, and key stakeholders to search for opportunities for cost reductions.

2. Where opportunities exist, use consensus criteria to define a standard of care.
3. Coach physicians in "discernment," the process of determining whether the standard is appropriate for treating a given patient.
4. Evaluate the aggregated outcomes of multiple applications of discernment so that everyone involved can understand whether the standard is being applied properly.
5. Intervene as needed to adjust the standard or its application.
6. Implement the standard.

To begin implementing its recommendations, IHI set up what it called an "appropriate use prototyping community." IHI had previously had great success using prototyping communities—in which "all teach; all learn"[20]— to spread quality initiatives. Some of the most notable of these communities developed the "ICU bundles" that dramatically decreased the incidence of ventilator-associated pneumonia in critical-care units[21] and decreased the incidence of sepsis (severe infection) from central venous catheters.[22]

IHI believed it could use the same type of framework for its appropriate-use prototyping community. But right from the start, there were problems. Whereas no medical institution has philosophical or practical objections to striving for better quality of care, the goal of reducing healthcare costs to patients carries with it the corollary of reducing revenues to organizations. So IHI found it unexpectedly difficult to recruit institutions even from the population that had successfully taken part in other improvement collaborative communities. Typically, IHI had at least a dozen institutions in any collaborative project; despite a vigorous recruiting effort, this time it was able to enroll only eight. Two dropped out almost immediately; the six remaining institutions, including the Palo Alto Medical Foundation, tried, through a series of in-person and telephone conversations, to use the prototyping process and the framework of the IHI white paper to develop local projects to see if specialty-care costs could be reduced by developing standards of care.

THE PROTOTYPING COMMUNITY

The six institutions involved in the prototyping community were different in structure. Three were large, multi-specialty medical groups: Advocate Physician Partners in Chicago, Illinois; HealthPartners Medical Group in Minneapolis, Minnesota; and Palo Alto Medical Foundation in Palo Alto, California. Two were smaller medical groups: Providence Medical Group in Portland, Oregon (a group of Primary Care physicians), and Tria Orthopedic Center in Minneapolis, Minnesota (a single specialty group practice). Huntington Hospital (North Shore–Long Island Jewish Health System) in Huntington, New York, is an academic institution. The small number of institutions and their differences in structure made it difficult to spread innovations among them.

One common theme that did emerge was a sense that medical groups of every size and constitution were at a disadvantage when negotiating with the physicians who provide them with specialty care. For many of the medical groups in the prototyping community, specialists were not an integral part of the group; rather, they were independent contractors who provided contracted services to the group. It was not uncommon for a medical group to be contracted with only one specialist or one group of specialists for a particular specialty; leaders of the medical groups worried that if they offended the specialty groups in some way, the specialists would no longer contract with them for services. And how could they not offend them? Because the specialists knew more about their work than the physicians running the prototyping community, how could these non-specialists credibly mandate that specialists change their behavior around appropriate use?

When PAMF joined the appropriate use prototyping community in 2009, we were already well along in our own variation-reduction program, which makes the physician the key role in the process. The changes in health-care practices we were making were something that physicians ourselves were doing. The IHI framework, in contrast, approached its project as something the organization was imposing on physicians. This conceptual disagreement was perhaps the most difficult and contentious issue in the prototyping community.

PAMF had tried this "top-down" approach throughout the heyday of managed care in the 1990s and found that we did not get the results we had hoped for. Because the Managed Care Department at PAMF was still responsible for determining whether to approve a test or procedure for patients with HMO insurance, I had begun working with the specialties to create local Managed Care clinical guidelines to replace the vague national guidelines that frequently offered little substantive guidance but set the medical director against the physician who actually saw the patient. Having already experienced the failure of the top-down approach, PAMF had decided that a grassroots, physician-led, bottom-up process was more promising. We felt it important not to substitute the judgment of the Managed Care medical director for the judgment of the physician who actually saw the patient. But the senior medical group leaders in the prototyping community who favored the top-down approach believed that letting their physicians determine their own appropriate-use projects was a failure of leadership. They already knew where the high-dollar over-utilization was occurring, and they were determined to do something about it. But while I had no doubt that these medical group leaders did understand where in their institutions the over-utilization was occurring, I couldn't see how their new plan was any different from previous efforts to impose managed care on physicians. Those efforts had done little more than alienate all the physicians involved.

The IHI prototyping community played itself out over about a nine-month period; unfortunately little was accomplished by its end in June 2010. To date, IHI has not made any sustained effort to again tackle the third arm of the triple aim with regard to specialty care; I suspect this type of effort will not yield results until institutions recognize that allowing unnecessary care has its own costs.

PAMF AT IHI

Meanwhile, PAMF's own efforts were bearing fruit, and IHI began to recognize them. At the December 2009 conference, our variation-reduction team had been allowed only a poster session to discuss our pilot project. For the meeting the next December, our proposal was granted presentation time.

When our team met with conference organizers the night before our talk and asked to see the space in which we would present, an organizer said, "We've been having difficulty finding a room for you." Looking at one another in surprise, we asked, "Why?" The response: "So many people signed up to hear your presentation that we had to find a bigger room." More than 800 people came to hear our findings the next day. After the talk, people lined up to ask questions about how they could start their own variation-reduction programs; we seemed to be answering questions almost as long as it had taken us to give the talk. For the 2011 conference, we didn't even have to submit a presentation; the organizers invited us to come back and provide an update on the success of our variation-reduction program.

What is it that PAMF is doing? How did it come about?

CHAPTER 3

The Inefficiency of "Efficiency"

PAMF took our first steps along the path to variation reduction in 2005, when our parent organization, Sutter Health, signed a contract with the Aetna Health Plan to bring "efficiency" to our healthcare delivery system. Aetna had partnered with a company called Symmetry to analyze claims data to develop what it called an efficiency index to rate individuals and groups of physicians.

Why did Sutter Health want this physician-specific cost data? It wanted to be a more cost-efficient provider. As a hospital system, it could influence facility cost of care by becoming more efficient operationally, but it had no way to affect cost of care controlled by its physicians. The first step in trying to influence physician-controlled cost of care was to obtain valid data on each physician. Sutter Health had a lot of interest in getting this kind of information. It was so interested, in fact, that it agreed to do something in contracting with Aetna that it had refused to do with any other health plan: tier the network.

TIERING A NETWORK

Health plans such as Aetna like the idea of a tiered physician network, which creates economic incentives for patients to see health plan–approved physicians. A health plan typically tiers its network by assigning a rating to each doctor or medical group according to some specified criteria. The top tier includes those physicians who have earned a "gold star," having made the grade according to those criteria. All other physicians fall into a second tier. A patient who chooses to see a gold-star physician has a lower out-of-pocket expense than a patient who chooses to see a lower-tier physician.

19

The beauty of network tiering from the health plan's point of view is that it side-steps the issue of healthcare rationing. It doesn't have to restrict a patient's access to more expensive physicians; patients themselves decide if they want to spend more out of pocket to continue to see their favorite physicians.

AETNA'S BLACK BOX

The second thing that Aetna brought to the table was episode treatment groups (ETGs). By using Symmetry's proprietary computer program, Aetna could collect two essential types of data: it could establish which physician was responsible for a given patient's care and it could risk-adjust the population for co-morbid conditions. If an organization can track who is responsible for the care of each patient, it can gather actionable data: an administrator can go to a physician and say, "These are the patients you took care of," a point from which a conversation can begin about clinical variation. Without this kind of attribution model, the data are too general; every physician can plausibly think, "The problem is with the next guy, not me."

The second issue, that of co-morbid conditions, is important especially when the number of patients in the population is small: clinically warranted variation may exist if, for example, one physician's panel of patients has more diabetics than another physician's panel. (Because diabetes is a co-morbid condition for most clinical episodes, the cost of surgery for a diabetic patient is appropriately greater than the cost to care for a patient without diabetes.) During the managed care boom, health plans that tried to present cost data frequently got pushback from the physicians, who argued "my patients are sicker than average," and "my patients have more co-morbid conditions and that's why their costs are higher." With the data supplied by ETGs, Symmetry's analysts would be able to control for co-morbidity.

According to the contract Sutter signed with Aetna in 2005, every medical group in Sutter would be listed as "efficient" for the first two years. Starting in the third year, Aetna would award gold-star status only to those groups that were efficient based on the criteria in the Aetna efficiency index.

The idea was that Aetna would provide Sutter with baseline information fairly quickly so groups could act to improve their efficiency before the tiered ratings appeared. Unfortunately, it took Aetna almost a half year to get the information to Sutter, and then additional time to deliver it to the various Sutter affiliates. PAMF didn't receive the information until the beginning of 2006.

COST NOT EFFICIENCY

When I received the first set of efficiency data in January 2006, I took one look at it and became upset. PAMF has three regions: Palo Alto, Camino, and Santa Cruz. Within the Camino region, where I principally worked at the time, Aetna had provided only grouped data for the physicians in nine specialty departments. Four of the nine specialties were initially deemed efficient; the other five were inefficient.

I had already been feeling uneasy about the prospect of using the terms "efficient" and "inefficient" to describe network physicians, or their departments, because the words carry such a heavy emotional load. But when I finally got a look at the elements that went into creating Aetna's efficiency index, I realized that the term itself was an intolerable misnomer. "Efficiency" implies both effectiveness of evaluation and quality of outcome. But the Aetna efficiency index was really just a measure of how expensive a physician group was in comparison to an unspecified and unknown control group.

ARE THE DATA WRONG?

My first reaction—which was similar to that of most other physicians faced with data like this—was to say, "This data is wrong; it's an unfair representation of our ability to care for patients." How could I justify imposing this type of ranking on my colleagues? But when my initial anger passed, I had a moment of clarity: if the contracts for our services were identical for all nine of these departments, why were some departments able to earn the efficiency rating while others were not? They all were getting paid the same rate for services. Something was a little strange.

When I looked more closely at the data, I found that the efficiency index was made on the basis of very small numbers of patients—so small that Aetna didn't have data enough to analyze the care provided by individual physicians, which is why it had aggregated its ratings on the departmental level. With such a small patient population, a single instance of unusually expensive care could brand an entire department inefficient for an entire reporting period. OK, but why did Aetna have so little data? It was because Aetna insurance covered less than 10% of our patient population.

These small numbers made it very difficult for me to believe Aetna's rankings, much less want to talk to individual physicians about why they or their departments were "inefficient." So I decided to try to replicate the Aetna data-gathering process using *all* of the patients in the Camino region of PAMF—in effect beginning a second, parallel project. We would analyze not a handful of patients per specialist, but hundreds of patients, and so be able to focus our analysis on individual physicians.

In an effort to move beyond Aetna's focus on physician "inefficiency," I began talking about our own cost-cutting or cost-reduction, or affordability project, but my colleagues felt that the terms were too much about money and not enough about quality. I appreciated their criticisms and became acutely aware of the importance of choosing nonjudgmental terminology to shape our conversations. I noticed how many of the terms used for the issue and its solutions, in both the medical and popular literature, negatively prejudge physicians' work before any conversation (or analysis) begins: terms like "waste," "overuse," "rationing," "death panels," "ineffective care," and "non-beneficial technologies." Even less-accusatory formulations, such as "promoting appropriate care," or "optimizing clinical value to patients," or "improving content of care," begin by assuming that physicians' pre-intervention decisions are wrong.

CHAPTER 4

Variation Reduction

In July 2006, I sent a memo to Camino president Rich Slavin detailing the parallel project, calling it the "variation-reduction project." We have used that term ever since. I think that the phrase "variation reduction" stuck for three reasons. First, it's nonjudgmental. I knew I needed to engage my physician colleagues to succeed in the project, and I was determined not to initiate any meeting handicapped by other physicians' beliefs that I was prejudging them. Second, the term accurately describes what I intended to do. Unwarranted clinical variation decreases value to patients by increasing cost and exposing them to unnecessary risk. Reducing variation increases that value. Third, "reduction" does not mean "elimination." Some variation will always be warranted; individual physicians must retain the freedom to use our own clinical judgment to make the best decisions for our patients, whether or not that treatment varies from the norm.

THE PREHISTORY OF VARIATION REDUCTION

In reaction to the limitations of the Aetna data (and the dubious wisdom of drawing conclusions from it), I became consumed with the idea that PAMF should make physician data-gathering a normal and integral part of every meeting between physician and patient.

I think that my preoccupation with data, the benefits of its careful analysis, and the sorrows of ignoring its lessons dates from early in my career as a pulmonologist, when I was taking care of a lot of patients in a critical-care unit. The neurosurgeons at our institution decided that they would try a regimen called barbiturate coma for patients who had sustained head trauma and were unconscious. The theory was that by putting the patient into a deep, pharmacologically induced coma, you could reduce the damage to the brain from the head injury. The barbiturate-coma regimen required that the patient be intubated, placed on a mechanical ventilator, and monitored extremely closely.

Four of the five neurosurgeons in our institution actively promoted this treatment; the fifth went along reluctantly, reasoning that the treatment was costly, untested, and dangerous, and that the small potential for improvement that it offered was outweighed by its risks. Each time a new head-trauma case was admitted to the critical-care unit, the nurses would dash around getting ready for the institution of the barbiturate-coma regimen. When the reluctant neurosurgeon was on call, he tried in vain to hold back this tidal wave of activity; the nurses disapproved of his efforts, making clear their opinion that he was giving substandard care in comparison to the other neurosurgeons.

After a year, a review of the data showed that the barbiturate-coma regimen had increased both cost and risk but had not improved outcomes. However, although the reluctant neurosurgeon had been proven correct, his colleagues shrugged off the evidence, moving on—equally enthusiastically—to the next new thing. Without regard to the clear results of the data analysis, the nursing staff continued to judge the reluctant neurosurgeon as substandard. He eventually left the institution, and left it poorer for his absence.

VARIATION REDUCTION 0.1

When I approached Aetna with my idea of gathering data from every encounter between physician and patient, it was cooperative in my quest— Aetna really was interested in helping me learn what data to gather and how to understand it—and gave me free access to its data-analysis company, Symmetry, and the development of its efficiency ratings. I was able to see what kinds of diagnoses Symmetry was including in these groupings. I was able to see how a specific co-morbid condition would weight a particular case more or less severe. With the help of a statistician, I determined that with our higher numbers, we would not need to use Symmetry's proprietary ETGs, which were developed for dealing with small numbers of patients. (With a large enough group of patients, all specialists are statistically likely to see about the same number of patients with co-morbid conditions as their colleagues.)

Using Aetna's nine-specialty framework, I ran the all-patient data for Camino. Our business office already maintained a data warehouse of encounters, one of which was generated every time a Camino physician saw a patient. For each encounter, the physician entered the type and level of service as well as the diagnosis. Initially these encounters were paper records sent to the business office to be entered into the computer system so bills could be generated. Office schedules were reconciled against these encounters so that missing reports could be entered.

With the help of one of our business analysts, I learned how to export information from the data warehouse to an Access database I could use to generate reports I could show to the physicians.

The first specialty I looked at was Ear, Nose, and Throat (ENT). Because Camino had only five ENT physicians, the ENT Department was small enough for me to gather the data easily, yet big enough to show variation. The Aetna data had suggested that chronic sinusitis was a good topic to look at, so as a first run at the data, I queried the database for all Camino patients with ENT encounters coded for chronic sinusitis. Then I totaled the charges by physician. I did find obvious differences among the five physicians on total charges, but I knew I couldn't present the data as they stood because two of the ENT physicians didn't work full time.

Although I considered dividing the total charges by the physicians' FTE status, I eventually decided to normalize the data by using a different metric: number of office visits for chronic sinusitis. I reasoned that the more office visits for chronic sinusitis an ENT physician logged, the more patients with chronic sinusitis the physician was seeing. So I created the metric of ENT charges for chronic sinusitis per 100 office visits for chronic sinusitis.

As shown in Figure 2, even after normalizing the metric, data from the five ENT physicians showed considerable variation in how they treated chronic sinusitis. When I shared the data with the ENT physicians, they were surprised and intrigued. They decided to work as a group to implement a best practice to reduce the variation.

I performed this kind of analysis for all nine of the Camino specialty groups, refining my methods as I learned. For example, it turned out that my decision to use number of office visits as a way to normalize data created a

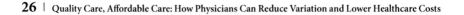

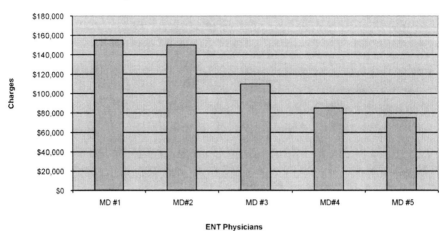

FIGURE 2. First variation-reduction graph on total charges for chronic sinusitis; normalized by number of office visits for chronic sinusitis.

result that was still problematic, because new physicians typically see more new patients than established specialists, and those new patients typically need more extensive workups than patients with chronic diseases. My office-visit metric could cause me to interpret warranted clinical variation as unwarranted.

Eight of the nine specialty groups reacted to the data by eventually deciding to develop best practices to reduce variation. By the end of 2007, when Aetna released its second set of metrics (again, using data only from the patients it insured), those eight departments had become efficient by Aetna's criteria. This result so pleased Aetna that it awarded the gold-star rating to all four divisions of PAMF and all of our specialty departments.

However, PAMF is only one of five Sutter Health medical groups; Aetna could not persuade the other Sutter groups to work with its data and soon abandoned both the project and the concept of tiering the network based on efficiency ratings.

VARIATION REDUCTION 1.0

If in the end, Aetna's project was a failure, PAMF's was not. The data we learned to develop at Camino gave us the ability to systematically examine individual healthcare decisions made by specialists in a 21st-century update of Jack Wennberg's work in Vermont.

In early 2008, PAMF experienced a significant reorganization: the three independent medical groups (Palo Alto Medical Clinic, Camino Medical Group, and Santa Cruz Medical Group) that had formed the original foundation integrated into a single organization. (The new organization's official name is the Palo Alto Foundation Medical Group, but people continue to know it as PAMF.) The integration of the three historic medical groups was necessary to benefit from economies of scale available only to large organizations. In addition, the new organization would be able to promote a consistent patient experience in the communities we serve.

This change had a profound effect on the Managed Care Department and our work on variation reduction. Where earlier I had been responsible for just the Camino Medical Group, now I oversaw the work of the new organization's more than 1000 physicians. In May 2008, the leadership at PAMF established affordability as a key goal for the new organization. (A second initiative was the redesign of Primary Care using lean principles.)

The success of the Camino pilot project started a number of balls rolling. PAMF leadership saw the variation-reduction process as a way to become more affordable. Leadership of PAMF's parent, Sutter Health, saw that giving data to physicians could change their behavior. Both organizations wanted to try to spread this work throughout the Sutter system. The PAMF Board set a goal that all specialty departments would have three variation-reduction projects up and running by the end of 2009, accepting my recommendation that it leave it up to its physicians to choose their own projects. The board also agreed that my refined data-collecting procedures were "good enough" and that PAMF would put its development time and money into training physicians to become variation-reduction champions.

In October 2008, I met with Dr. Laurel Trujillo, head of the quality committee for the Palo Alto division, to discuss how to scale the affordability initiative to all physicians in the new organization. There has always been some tension at PAMF between the people who work in quality and the people who work in managed care. But the leadership of both departments knew that both affordability and quality were necessary for PAMF to meet the needs of our community. We needed a way to merge the need to reduce cost and the need to improve quality.

Because I was the managed care medical director and had initiated the variation-reduction project, the preliminary work had been done as an extension of my department. For convenience, the expanded project would continue under managed care. But we both felt that for variation reduction to be embraced by the majority of our colleagues, we had to make it clear that variation reduction isn't primarily a managed care–type cost-cutting initiative. Rather, it's an issue of quality of care and the path to increased value for our patients. To that end, we decided that the variation-reduction project would report to the quality-improvement steering committee.

In the three years that I'd been working on variation reduction, it had been mostly a solo enterprise. Now Dr. Trujillo and I agreed that we would create a formal variation-reduction steering group. The steering group would develop and lead a team of physicians and data analysts to spread the variation reduction throughout all of PAMF. Dr. Trujillo was based in the Palo Alto division; I was based in Camino. To make sure that our project would be a foundation-wide effort, we needed to recruit a physician from Santa Cruz. Dr. Wendi Knapp, a hospitalist, was recommended by Santa Cruz leadership; Dr. Knapp accepted the nomination. Our steering group was now well-balanced geographically as well as by function: as a pulmonologist, I brought the specialist viewpoint; Dr. Trujillo brought the Primary Care point of view; and Dr. Knapp brought insight into hospital procedures.

Early on, the variation-reduction steering group made several important decisions. The first was that we would continue to focus on our specialist colleagues, not Primary Care physicians, for two reasons. First, the Primary Care physicians were already busy with another affordability-related project whose goal was to streamline the role of the Primary Care physicians and enable to them to work with increased numbers of patients. Second, all of our data suggested that the major opportunities for cost reduction—a necessary early "win"—lay with the specialists.

Our second decision was that to make our comparative data better, we would analyze only new patients seen by a specialist for a particular clinical problem. The initiating encounter for data collection would be when the patient saw the specialist for a new consultation. That decision clarified and simplified our data collection and analysis: we would not have to adjust our findings for varying levels of maturity of the physician/patient relationship.

Our third decision was to affirm that while data gathering was necessary, it was a secondary consideration; the discussion about the standard was more important. Our goal was cultural change, a change that would engage physicians at a grassroots level to think about increasing value to the patient by increasing quality and decreasing cost.

Finally, we agreed that we did not need to experiment any more. Instead of more pilot projects, we would go into production: the board had set the goal of three variation-reduction projects per specialty by the end of 2009, and if we were going to meet that goal we needed to get started now.

The three members of the variation-reduction steering group set a goal to meet with physicians in every one of the 22 targeted specialties in PAMF by the end of the first quarter of 2009. (As it turned out, both the board's goal and the steering group's goals were a stretch. It took us until the end of 2010—almost two years—before we were able to meet with every one of the specialty departments.)

We devised a formula for these kickoff meetings and the projects they would initiate. In the first part of a kickoff meeting, we would present the case for why PAMF needed to become more affordable. Next, we would explain the idea of increasing value through reducing unwarranted variation. Next, we would summarize the methodology we used to derive the data that would reveal the variation. Finally, we would show the specialists their specific data and invite them to create their own variation-reduction projects.

After identifying the focus for a variation project, the specialists' first task would be to develop a standard of care. We classified those projects into three buckets. A project under discussion was one that did not yet have an agreed-upon standard. An active project had a set standard, but no follow-up data. A mature project had both the set standard and its follow-up data.

The first specialty physicians who were willing to meet as a single, foundation-wide group were the Urologists. Nine Urologists comprised the new joint Urology Department: four from Palo Alto, three from Camino, and two from Santa Cruz. Two of the Urologists, Jim Bassett and Arnie Aigen, were also medical group board members; their support of the variation-reduction project was key. In retrospect it was fortunate that these two leaders were part of our first integrated project and were themselves interested in affordability and variation reduction. They were key in getting their specialty and the group as a whole to participate in the project. While I'd like to say that I knew I needed to seek out these urologist/board member thought leaders, in fact their presence was happenstance. Later, the steering group purposefully sought board members and other leaders to get them actively involved with variation reduction.

CHAPTER 5

Our Results

By the end of December 2008, the variation-reduction team had met with the departments of Urology, Allergy, Ophthalmology, Dermatology, Oncology, and Sleep Medicine. Allergy was the first to create and implement a standard of care. The variation-reduction team had shown the eight allergists data establishing that the most common reason patients consult them is for allergic rhinitis. The data showed significant variation among the allergists in the charges generated for this condition, ranging from a high of $1,700 to a low of $750 per patient over a one-year period.

When the variation-reduction team and the allergists went over the data together, we realized that the driving factor of the variation in cost was the number of skin tests ordered for a new patient. Some allergists performed as few as 20 skin tests; others did as many as 100. The allergists searched the medical literature and found no evidence-based standard for the number of skin tests required to diagnose allergic rhinitis. Based on the types of allergens in our local area, they decided on a standard of 40 skin tests. In the five months before the new standard was put into effect, the eight allergists had seen 1220 new patients for allergic rhinitis. In the five months after the standard went into effect, they saw 1419 new patients for the same condition. The average charge per patient decreased by $360, with a total savings of $200,000 in the five-month period. What's more, by creating a standard of care and eliminating unwarranted tests, they decreased costs while increasing quality of care. Patients who had formerly undergone too few skin tests received better diagnoses and patients who had undergone too many tests avoided an unnecessary number of the often painful pinpricks. These were the findings we presented at the December 2009 IHI poster session.

By October 2009, we'd held kickoff meetings with 20 of the 22 specialties; by the end of the year, we had 14 active projects including glaucoma follow-up care, the use of white-cell stimulators in breast-cancer chemotherapy, and the optimal number of epidural ejections for low-back pain.

By April 2010, five of the active projects had matured to the point that we could report the results. In each of the specialties (Urology, Physiatry, General Surgery, Ophthalmology, and Allergy), significant reduction in unwarranted variation occurred, decreasing the cost to the patient without loss of quality.

How did we know that no quality was lost? For each of these projects, we tracked what we called a balance quality measure to complement the cost measure and ensure that quality was being maintained. In the oncology project, which reduced the use of the white-blood-cell stimulators, for example, we tracked the incidence of serious infections among patients with breast cancer who were treated with chemotherapy. The incidence remained the same before and after the institution of the standard.

Total savings were $2.9 million.

By October 2010, the number of mature projects had reached 15 and the savings were $8.3 million. By November 2011, we had 20 mature projects, 11 active projects, and 13 projects under discussion, with a combined total savings of $17.1 million. By the end of 2012, we had 62 projects in total: 24 mature, 18 active, and 20 under discussion. Our cumulative savings were $31.3 million.

✦ ✦ ✦

Our success has bred its own problems. For the first few years of the variation-reduction program, I had analyzed all the data myself. Beginning in 2010, demands for data increased faster than I could keep up with them. Some projects or potential projects began to slip through the cracks. Fortunately, the organization recognized the benefits of the program and invested more money into the project to build up the team. We added three new physician champions, who worked 20% of their time on variation reduction. We hired a full-time analyst to help with the demands for data. Finally, to coordinate all these efforts, we hired a part-time project manager (later promoted to project director). That's the team we have today.

Our success with specialty variation reduction also created unanticipated discontent in our more than 500 Primary Care physicians. Members of the Primary Care leadership came to see me in mid-2010, demanding that we start a Primary Care–based variation-reduction project. At first I told them that it was out of the scope of the project, but they were insistent, and I relented when they said that if we didn't do it with them, they would do it themselves. (It took me a while to realize that they were forcing on me what I actually wanted: physicians proactively taking the reins to reduce variation.)

The Primary Care physicians wanted to look at the treatment of hypertension, the most common chronic medical problem that Primary Care sees. The data challenges were significant. Our medical group treats 120,000 adult patients with hypertension, for a total of more than 600,000 office visits per year. Those patients are seen by more than 300 Primary Care providers (PCPs).

When we tried to use our usual variation-reduction methodology of starting data collection with the first visit of a new patient for the specific malady, we quickly realized that it wouldn't work in this case, because many new patient visits to PCPs were not equivalent to the new-consult visit of the specialists; instead, a new patient visit was more typically because the patient had changed insurance and needed a new PCP. Each of those patients came with a list of chronic problems that frequently included hypertension. For this project, then, we adopted an attribution model that surveyed all the physicians a patient saw and designated as the patient's PCP the physician with the most office visits resulting in a diagnosis of hypertension. In the initial data sets we looked only at office visits, laboratory, and imaging encounters with a hypertension diagnosis attached. Later we would add in pharmacy data.

Figure 3 shows physician variation in the average charge per patient to treat hypertension. When we superimposed the percentage of patients whose hypertension was under treatment, we found no relationship between the amount that PCPs charged and the degree to which their patients' blood pressure was under control. This discrepancy was a sharp wake-up call to most of the Primary Care providers.

In 2011, PAMF leadership had visited ThetaCare in Wisconsin to get a firsthand look at a medical group using lean management techniques (sometimes called the Toyota production model).[23] Subsequently, PAMF incorporated those techniques in the Primary Care redesign project, so the variation-reduction team decided to adapt to the model by holding a

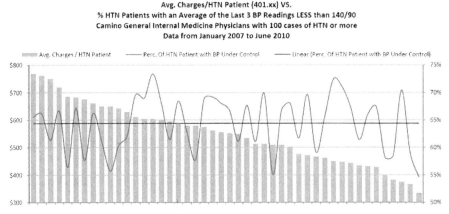

FIGURE 3. Cost of care for hypertension by individual provider. Each bar is the average charge per patient for that provider; the line indicates the average number of patients with blood pressure under control for each PCP.

"kaizen" event on hypertension. (In Japanese, "kai" means to change or to correct and "zen" means good. A "change for the good" describes this event well.) Typically a kaizen event is a way to change a factory production process but this event was to be a clinical kaizen; the goal was to change the way Primary Care providers managed hypertension.

In January 2011, Primary Care leadership and the variation-reduction team brought 40 people involved in Primary Care together for a two-day kaizen. Twenty-one were physicians; they had been asked to survey their colleagues on how they treated hypertension and bring the results to the meeting. To ensure a broad range of viewpoints, we also invited medical assistants, nurses, a data analyst, and three patients. The large group was divided into four work groups: diagnosis, treatment, follow up, and innovation, each of which was tasked with developing a standard work procedure, to be completed in the next month. The diagnosis group, for example, was to review the evidence and practice on how blood pressure was checked at PAMF and then make recommendations to run a blood pressure measurement pilot project. A month later, we held a second, one-day meeting to hear the reports of the groups and to define the hypertension standard: uniform measurement of blood pressure, standardized documentation in the electronic medical record, agreed-upon treatment, and planned and scripted follow-up care.

It took four months to train 312 PAMF medical assistants and nurses on the new standard method for taking blood pressure. In August 2011, variation-reduction team members and Primary Care leadership began a three-month process to visit all 30 Primary Care sites to roll out the standard. By the end of 2012, implementation of the new hypertension standard had saved $2.4 million. During this first full year, we reduced the average number of visits for hypertension from 1.6 visits per year to 1.4. While this reduction might seem modest, it affected 25,000 patients and freed up 5000 visit slots so that other patients could be seen. With the standard, the percentage of patients in control rose from 77% to 78.3%—an additional 613 patients who had blood pressure under control, reducing their risk for heart attack, stroke, and kidney failure. The standard not only saved dollars and improved quality of care, it also improved Primary Care access: a triple play! And this example has repeated over and over at PAMF: small, incremental changes that save significant amounts of money, benefit our existing patients, and open up our care to the community.

In November 2012, PAMF's leadership met to discuss the specific issue of how we would continue to reduce total cost of care. During the brainstorming part of the meeting, we listed all our current programs that affect cost of care as well as new programs we might want to implement. The next part of the process was to rank the programs, choosing the initiatives that the group would concentrate on over the next year. Each of the 15 members was to vote for three programs, which meant that any program could gain a maximum possible total of 15 votes. I voted for variation reduction, as did one other person. And only one program—the variation-reduction program—received only two votes. While I sat there, stunned, a senior leader (who later told me that he was the other vote) said,"I don't understand why variation reduction got so few votes. It's the only program we have that we know works." Others replied that they knew that; they just supposed that the program was already so far along it needed no special attention: variation reduction is so entrenched in PAMF, it's simply thought of as the way we practice medicine. In many ways, that's the place to be in an organization, so entrenched that the program is taken as a given. The first part of this book explained how PAMF got here; Part II describes what a physician, physician leader, or a physician group administrator needs to do to bring their organization to the same point.

Part II:

Changing Minds, Changing Practices

CHAPTER 6

Why Bother?

At the 2010 Group Practice Improvement Network (GPIN) conference, a national meeting of large multi-specialty medical groups, our team gave a plenary presentation on variation reduction. After I finished my part, someone snarked from the back of the room, "Did the CEOs of the insurance companies you deal with give you a nice Christmas present?" What my questioner was asserting, in essence, was that because the healthcare payment mechanism hasn't changed yet, the only thing variation reduction is accomplishing right now is to increase insurance companies' profits and decrease our own.

And there's some truth to that. The major beneficiary of our cost savings so far is, or could be, insurance companies, because if we spend less on a patient's treatment, the patient's insurance company gets to keep the extra profit; there's no assurance that a reduction in utilization will be reflected in a lower premium to patients. In fact, at a recent meeting of the California statewide pay-for-performance group, which included representatives of all the major state medical groups and health plans, we brought up this very issue: when our program achieves cost reductions, who gets to share in the savings? Most of the physicians at the meeting wanted some assurance from the plans that physician-instigated savings would be returned to the patients in lower premiums. The plans were not willing to make that commitment.

So why worry about total cost of care now?

In the "good old days" of managed care, when nearly half of PAMF's patients had HMO-type health insurance, it was obvious that controlling the total cost of care benefitted our medical group. The fewer HMO dollars PAMF spent, the more money our group could distribute to our physicians. Now that the number of patients with HMO insurance has dropped to less than 25% of our patient base, it's harder for PAMF's physicians to maintain the HMO ethic of controlling the cost of care.

Take, for example, physical therapy (PT). PAMF provides some PT services in-house but most are provided by outside PT providers, some of which contract with us, some of which do not. In the past, PAMF physicians referred most of our patients with HMO insurance to our contracted providers, which in turn discounted our HMO-patient rate because they knew that we would also send them our patients with fee-for-service insurance (for whom they charged higher prices).

But HMO reimbursement has been stagnant for some time now, and PT providers who work with HMOs have tried to minimize their peripheral expenses (for example, by using more aides and fewer certified physical therapists) in order to maintain their essential services. So although PAMF physicians have stayed with the contracted PT providers for patients with HMO insurance, they've begun to refer their patients with fee-for-service insurance to non-contracted PT providers who provide more personalized care at—of course—a higher price. (In fact, most of the boutique PT providers in our area charge 30% more than the contracted HMO providers, although it's unclear if this increased cost results in better outcomes.)

So what happened when our physicians started referring patients with fee-for-service insurance to the non-contracted PT providers? The contracted providers reacted by dropping their discounts for patients with HMO insurance. The overall effect was to increase the total cost of care for patients with HMO insurance, which increases premiums to employers, lessens the number of patients with HMO insurance, decreases the physicians' HMO ethic (and payments), and increases the cost of care: a vicious downward spiral.

While not as obvious, market forces can create similar conditions for patients with fee-for-service insurance, too. When a large employer removes a high-priced medical group from its network, and the number of the group's patients with fee-for-service insurance decreases, its physicians tend to perform more procedures on the remaining patients to maintain the group's revenue. This physician practice increases the total cost of care; to control rising costs, other employers narrow their own networks to providers willing to accept lower reimbursements or they increase out-of-pocket expenses for their employees. This employer response decreases the number of patients seen by physicians, who increase utilization or price for the remaining patients; again, a vicious downward spiral. While this second type of downward spiral never occurred at PAMF, the possibility was always there.

Market forces—not how many patients with HMO or fee-for-service insurance a group has—necessitate controlling total cost of care no matter the form of physicians' reimbursement schemes. PAMF physicians, like many in the United States, get paid to take care of patients with both HMO and fee-for-service insurance. If you ask them whether they treat these two groups differently, the answer is an emphatic no, a plausible response because while PAMF is paid differently by the different types of insurance, it pays its individual physicians for productivity, generally measured by number of patients seen. (Even physicians who see only patients with HMO insurance are paid on productivity, albeit measured by the number of shifts worked rather than the number of patients seen.)

But this insistence is a bit of self-delusion on the part of most physicians: they say they don't treat patients based on the type of insurance they have, but in fact they do, as demonstrated by a steady increase in procedures done on patients with HMO insurance as opposed to the number of procedures done on patients with fee-for-service insurance. When I've asked our physicians to explain the difference, one of the frequent answers I hear is that they know that a patient with HMO insurance has no or little out-of-pocket expense, so there's a lower barrier for recommending the procedure.

Pay for *quantity* is the common pattern for most multi-specialty medical groups in the United States. Some groups have begun experimenting with different ways of compensating physicians that attempt to pay for value instead, measured by clinical outcomes, access to physicians, and/or patient satisfaction. But for now, because physicians are paid more when they do more, it's easy to see why the cost for healthcare continues to increase.

◆   ◆   ◆

The Palo Alto Medical Foundation is located in the San Francisco Bay area. This area is also the birthplace of the Kaiser Permanente system, which is one of the largest HMOs in the country. For HMOs like Kaiser, working to decrease the amount of unnecessary care makes both economic and ethical sense. When an HMO appropriately decreases utilization, patients benefit with increased quality of care at a lower cost.

Within the Kaiser system, reducing unnecessary care benefits everyone, including physicians. Outside of Kaiser or Kaiser-like systems, this is not the case. The only way a physician gets paid in the non-HMO setting is to provide a service to a patient. Doing less means reducing your income. In this way, the current reimbursement system incentivizes physicians to do more, not less, especially for patients insured by Medicare, the largest insurer in the United States, which has no pre-authorization process. A physician simply performs the service and bills Medicare for it. Whether the service is necessary is rarely the issue, just the fact that it was performed. So it's not surprising that Jack Wennberg and his team at Dartmouth found so much of Medicare's expenditures in the supply-sensitive bucket. Or that Atul Gawande, who found the Medicare-supported system of care in McAllen, Texas, oriented more toward maximizing physician revenues than caring for patient needs, worried that its focus on the business of healthcare would cease to be an outlier and instead become the norm.

The Kaiser system takes care of 30% to 40% of all the patients in the Bay area. It provides high-quality care by all objective standards and has high patient satisfaction. Because Kaiser is a fully integrated system where the entire spectrum of care, from hospital and ambulatory clinics to nursing homes and home care, is all in the same system, Kaiser achieves high quality at a lower premium than PAMF can offer. (PAMF, for the most part, uses hospitals that are not part of PAMF. These hospitals have their own financial goals, which are not necessarily in alignment with the PAMF goal of decreasing the total cost of care.) One of the restrictions that patients agree to when they sign up for Kaiser insurance is that they will seek care only from Kaiser physicians, and only at Kaiser facilities. So Kaiser patients aren't seen at PAMF.

PAMF does contract with Aetna, Anthem Blue Cross, Blue Shield, Cigna, HealthNet, and UnitedHealthcare, the six largest health plans other than Kaiser. Our contracts with the plans include all products: HMO, PPO, and, if available, the Medicare Advantage (or senior HMO) plans. These six companies represent all of our HMO business and 80% of our PPO business.

The HMO model of healthcare has been popular in Northern California. But over the last 10 years there's been a significant and persistent shift away from HMO plans to PPO plans. In the mid-1990s, nearly 50% of PAMF's patients had HMO insurance. But the managed care revolution of the 1990s was not well-received by patients. Audiences cheered when Helen Hunt's character in the 1997 movie *As Good as It Gets* curses her HMO insurance and the doctor in the film agrees. HMO flight increased with the creation of Health Savings Accounts (HSAs), which allowed patients to save pre-tax money to use to pay healthcare costs, and which were almost always linked to PPO insurance. By 2012, PAMF's HMO percentage had dropped to 20%.

Initially, HMO insurance was less expensive to the employer than PPO insurance; now the reverse is true: the smaller the pool of patients with HMO insurance got, the more expensive the plan became. HMO plans attracted patients with chronic problems because patients could budget how much per month they'd have to spend on healthcare, something they couldn't do with PPO insurance, where patients are responsible for more, and more unpredictable, out-of-pocket expense than if they have HMO plans.

In Silicon Valley, where PAMF is located, many of the high-tech companies are self-insured through Employee Retirement Income Security Act (ERISA) plans, which basically allow them to use insurance companies for administrative services only, reducing the overhead and profit that the health plans have added to the healthcare system without limiting networks or adding cost to the employee. Typically, self-insurance reduces the companies' healthcare expenditures by about 10%.

Three years ago, one of PAMF's largest participating employers was offering its employees three different HMOs (Kaiser and two commercial HMOs) plus a high-deductible PPO plan. At that point, Kaiser cost less than the other HMOs by about $50 per month. At that small a savings, most of the patients with HMO insurance chose to stay with one of the two commercial HMOs and remain with PAMF. A year later, the employer changed its insurance structure; the commercial HMOs increased their prices over Kaiser to about $100 per month. In response to the new price point, a significant number of employees switched to Kaiser even though it meant changing doctors and leaving PAMF. This year the employer narrowed its network by dropping the two commercial HMO plans as unaffordable. If employees wanted to see a PAMF physician, they would have to switch to the high-deductible PPO plan, which meant even more out-of-pocket expense for the employee.

What makes this example most striking is that the employer was Stanford University and Stanford Hospital. Stanford and the Palo Alto division of PAMF sit side by side. While the two organizations are totally separate, and their outpatient clinics compete for ambulatory care, each depends on the other. Stanford depends on PAMF to be a major referral source for tertiary care; PAMF uses the Stanford Hospital as its community hospital for much routine care such as delivering babies. Like PAMF, Stanford Hospital is not part of the Kaiser system, so by dropping the commercial HMOs, Stanford created a situation in which its own employees can no longer use the hospital where they work—let alone PAMF—if they want an HMO plan. Stanford as an employer is not willing to pay the price of Stanford as a provider!

◆ ◆ ◆

When employers self-insure, they can actually see where their healthcare dollars are spent. In addition, with the increase in high-deductible PPO plans, the employees as consumers of the healthcare can also see the billed costs of services provided. Under this system, it's our view that PAMF must be able to reduce healthcare costs so our participating employers will be less likely to move to less-expensive health plans such as Kaiser. Perhaps we can also win employers like Stanford back.

As it became clear that the market for healthcare was changing, and afford-ability was an area of vulnerability for PAMF, we knew that we needed to get going on affordability even before the reimbursement scheme changes. We needed to make our care more affordable for our patients, and we needed to increase the value to our patients. Now that we have solid data that we have been able to increase both affordability and value, we have begun to work with several health plans and employers in what we call "shared-savings arrangements," arrangements with self-insured employers that are interested in reducing their healthcare costs while maintaining the quality of care for their employees.

Basically, a shared-savings program is a fee-for-service/PPO-type health plan. Members of this health plan are not obligated to see any particular provider within the organization; they are not assigned to a Primary Care provider, nor is there any gatekeeping function. Using data from the insurance company, the medical group and the employer develop a budget for healthcare costs for that patient population, with the goal of reducing the overall healthcare expenditures by a certain percentage. If PAMF physicians meet the target, our group and the employer share the savings. This arrangement is similar in concept to the plans offered by Medicare Accountable Care Organizations (ACOs), but for patients with commercial insurance.

PAMF has two main levers that we can pull to become more affordable. The first lever is unit price: how much we charge for a particular test, visit, or procedure. The other lever is utilization: how often we do a given test, visit, or procedure. Unit price in a large multi-specialty group is not typically under the control of the individual physician. Instead, the management team sets what we call a "charge master" to standardize prices across the organization. Utilization, on the other hand, is directly controlled by the individual physician. Self-insured employers see the effect of changes in both unit price and utilization. Individual patients see only the effect of changes in unit price; it's hard for them to feel a change in utilization.

Indeed, it's hard even for individuals with backgrounds in healthcare to see the effect of changes in utilization. At a recent statewide pay-for-performance meeting, one of the committee members with a lot of experience in healthcare policy told me that he had just had his colon cancer–screening colonoscopy at PAMF, and while he had a great patient experience, he was shocked at the cost. He knew that he could get the procedure done elsewhere for less money, so what were we thinking?

I asked him when he was scheduled to come back for his next screening colonoscopy.

"Ten years," he replied.

"Find out the return rate on that lower-priced colonoscopy," I said. "I bet they'd have you coming back in five years." Taking the longer view, PAMF was more affordable—and far less uncomfortable—as anyone who has had a colonoscopy will tell you.

◆ ◆ ◆

Utilization of services is in the hands of the individual physicians. Variation reduction gives physicians a way to control utilization by open discussion of the clinical issues rather than some absolute rationing dictum imposed from above. Variation reduction and PAMF's commitment to quality are two of the reasons health plans and employers have been willing to start discussions on shared-savings models.

Developing a shared-savings program is not trivial. Enlisting the cooperation of all the parties involved in sharing data is difficult, not only because of patient-privacy issues, but also because of anti-trust issues. In developing a budget for a given group of patients, you have to know which patients the medical group is going to be responsible for. The attribution process, by its very nature, is retrospective, which is markedly different from the prospective HMO attribution process. In an HMO, patients have to choose which medical group they will use as their primary medical group; from that moment on, they need to access all their care through that primary medical group. This, of course, is one of the major objections to the HMO system in general. Patients who choose PPO-type insurance do so because they want the freedom to go to any provider within their network of physicians.

In a shared-savings arrangement, we not only need to develop a budget for the employer's healthcare costs, we also need to agree on the appropriate attribution model. A patient who has seen one of our Primary Care physicians in the previous 18 months is considered our patient when we are looking at a shared-savings program. Patients seen by Primary Care physicians not associated with our group are not counted in our cost to the employer even if we provide some specialty care for that patient. Similarly, a patient who sees a PAMF Primary Care physician is counted within our cost in the shared-savings arrangement even when the patient obtains specialty care from a non-PAMF physician.

An issue with this attribution model is that there's a third group of patients: the ones who see a specialist without first seeing any Primary Care physician at all. How we attribute these patients, and how big an effect they have on the total healthcare cost to the employer, is unclear at this point. The conventional wisdom is that establishing a patient with a Primary Care physician decreases total cost of care.

Another interesting new wrinkle in the attribution model is whether to attribute a patient to PAMF if the only contact is electronic. The vast majority of our patients use our My Health online service. Through this service, patients can have secure E-mail conversations with their physicians, check their medical records, schedule appointments, and even pay their bills. In a recent internal survey, Sutter Health looked at 40,000 patients seen by Primary Care physicians and found that 11% of the patients were attributed to their Primary Care provider only by such electronic contact. Our current thinking is that e-visits and other non–face-to-face encounters may become much more commonplace because patients like them and they allow us to provide care for the patient at a lower cost. The issue now is that our current attribution models do not take this type of encounter into account.

At PAMF, we think these shared-savings plans are the future of affordable healthcare because they align the incentives of both the provider and purchaser of healthcare. Most of PAMF's patients with PPO insurance are in employer self-insured plans. In that they're paying all the costs of healthcare, these self-insured employers are taking on the same role as the federal government takes with Medicare. These employers (and Medicare) are now able to see the effect of unnecessary care as it adds to their healthcare spend.

If the only way physicians are paid to care for patients is a fee-for-service model, then it stands to reason that physicians will continue to do more and more. When faced with the choice of doing nothing and not getting paid or doing something for which they will get paid, the choice is obvious. Shared-savings plans reinstate the aligned incentives of both the purchasers and providers of healthcare that were present in the HMO model but were lost when most patients switched to the fee-for-service model. Both purchaser and provider want high-quality care and both want to benefit from controlling the cost of care. A shared-savings plan gives the physician an incentive not only to avoid marginal procedures but also to participate in the work of variation reduction. Changing the reimbursement model will be key to bending the rising cost curve of healthcare.

◆ ◆ ◆

In this first chapter of Part II, I examined why medical groups should begin the work of variation reduction when structural incentives have not yet changed. The remaining chapters of this section discuss the transformations in thinking and practice necessary to implement a variation-reduction program. Chapter 7 engages the very real objections that physicians have to beginning such a program; Chapter 8 discusses the need to develop local physicians as the experts you rely on for clinical judgments. Chapter 9 examines the sources of variation in those judgments; Chapter 10 introduces the pillars of variation reduction, five principles our variation-reduction team developed as the foundation for beginning a variation-reduction program.

CHAPTER 7

Addressing Physicians' Concerns

R ecently I spoke about variation reduction at my medical school alma mater, the University of California, San Francisco. During the discussion period, I was pleased to hear that the Department of Medicine has instituted into its curriculum for training internists the effect of physician ordering on the total cost of patient care. For all the talk about patient-driven care, the physician is still the one to order the test, prescribe the medication, and perform the procedure. That's why physicians are at the center of variation reduction.

At PAMF, the Managed Care Department has been fairly successful in making the case to physicians that we need to be less expensive or we'll continue to lose market share. Every physician has had the personal experience of an increasing number of patients saying, "I just can't afford this. I have a high-deductible plan. I'm not going to do what you're recommending because it's too expensive."

Variation reduction is an attractive way for PAMF physicians to reduce costs while maintaining—and even increasing—quality of care. But with every specialty group the variation-reduction team has talked with, we've also found that our specialists have significant individual and organizational concerns about the process. To establish trust between the variation-reduction team and the specialists, we have had to address concerns about income, patient satisfaction, productivity, autonomy, and "cookbook medicine."

"WON'T THIS LOWER MY INCOME?"

Probably the first thing that occurs to most physicians when they hear about variation reduction is that it could reduce their incomes.

At PAMF, more than three-quarters of our revenue is from fee-for-service patient care. We pay most of our physicians based on a productivity system. The more they do, the more they make. (Certain specialties such as Radiology and the hospitalists are paid a salary; productivity is not taken into account. PAMF did not want to influence our radiologists to perform more procedures because unnecessary procedures expose patients to more radiation and potential harm. Similarly, we wanted avoid the potential conflict of interest that might arise by using a productivity-based compensation system to compensate hospitalists. When we started the hospitalist program, one goal was to reduce patients' length of stay in the hospital; paying a hospitalist more to keep a patient in the hospital was the wrong incentive.)

PAMF's experience with variation-reduction projects is that the physicians paid for doing more often end up creating standards of care that recommend doing less. Asking physicians to do less when they're paid for productivity can seem like asking them to act against their own self-interests. But that's not really the case.

Recently the variation-reduction team had a meeting with PAMF's hand surgeons, who were examining the treatment of carpal-tunnel syndrome. One surgeon—very outspoken, with a no-nonsense view of the world—said, "You know, this doesn't make any sense. We're just going to lose money. Why are we even thinking about doing this?"

I turned to him and said, "Do you have a waiting list?"

"Oh, yeah," he said, "but if you broke your hand, I'd see you today."

"Yeah, I understand if I broke my hand, you'd see me today," I said. "But suppose I just called your office and said, 'My hand hurts. How soon can I be seen?'"

And he said, "Well, probably two weeks."

And I said, "Probably three weeks!"

And he said, "Yeah, probably."

Would creating a standard of care really cost him money, I asked, or would it just improve his practice? "We know that one of the most common reasons patients come to see you is for carpal tunnel. Would it be better if we had a standard of care for carpal tunnel that everybody agreed on, that the Primary Care providers knew about, so they'd send you appropriate referrals, not the referrals that you don't really need to see? That they'd only send you patients who have already gone through physical therapy and a course of non-steroidal anti-inflammatory agents?"

And he said, "Well, yeah, because that's the first thing that I do with everybody anyway, and it's sort of a waste of my time."

And I said, "Exactly. If we can take out those unnecessary visits, and get you only the patients that you really need to see, what would happen?"

I could see the wheels turning.

What variation reduction does, basically, is remove productivity that's not appropriate and substitute productivity that is—seeing the next new patient. What would happen if we suddenly eliminated the backlog of new patients? Well, should that happen, some physicians' income might well decrease, but that's not likely to happen any time soon. Timely access to specialty care is a nationwide problem; variation reduction can help alleviate it.

"WON'T THIS SKEW MY STATS?

A second potential concern for physicians is fear that following a variation-reduction standard may decrease patient satisfaction. Patient satisfaction is one of the publicly reported quality measures in California, and self-initiated reports of patient satisfaction via social media, such as Yelp, are increasingly influential. At PAMF, we spend a lot of time and energy trying to improve patient satisfaction. We survey patients frequently; each physician is rated by at least 30 separate encounters every year. In the patient-centric healthcare model, patient satisfaction is one of the main measures of how well a physician is doing, and improving patient satisfaction is one of the main goals of our medical group. So physicians are loathe to make any changes that would decrease patient satisfaction.

Take the example of low back pain, which is one of the most common reasons patients come to see a Primary Care provider. The PCP has to be concerned not only with making an accurate diagnosis but managing patient expectations. Some patients come into the office convinced that they need an MRI—they heard from friends or relatives that if you don't have an MRI, something terrible might be missed. Whether or not the patient meets the standard for low-back-pain imaging, it's easier for a busy PCP to just order the MRI than try to manage the patient's expectations: refusing to order the MRI may increase the likelihood that that patient will rate the physician poorly on a satisfaction survey.

A discussion with a patient about why it's not appropriate to do something frequently takes longer than a discussion of why to do something. In this Internet-savvy, information-glutted society, especially in Northern California, patients frequently come in with their own diagnoses and their own decisions on a course of action. Going against the trend can be a difficult task for a physician. No wonder some physicians are uncomfortable with the variation-reduction process!

Our response to this concern is to say, "It's part of your job as a physician to educate your patients. If you just give patients unnecessary tests, are you doing the right thing for them?" Most of our physicians recognize the problem. They agree that it's not right to order unnecessary tests, but they have the issue of patient satisfaction in the front of their minds all the time.

I don't think our group really has come to a complete understanding of the interrelationship between variation reduction and patient satisfaction, and that conflict is evident in our reward system: while we do pay physicians for increasing patient satisfaction, we do not pay for increasing use of variation-reduction standards. It would not be surprising if individual physicians get the subliminal message that patient satisfaction is more important than variation reduction.

In fact, it is quite amazing how, for the most part, physicians at the Palo Alto Medical Foundation have accepted and worked toward the goals of variation reduction. Even though I have asked our board of directors to incentivize our physicians for participation in the variation-reduction projects, I have been unable to get anything more than funds to pay for the physician time spent at the committee meetings and, of course, food. The board has said that this project is something that we all need to do; it's the right thing. It's the board's opinion that we should do it without additional compensation. While I personally applaud this stance, it would be nice to reward some of the specialty groups who have gone above and beyond requirements to develop really far-reaching standards.

"WON'T THIS HURT MY PRODUCTIVITY?"

A third issue is that variation reduction appears to conflict with initiatives to increase productivity. Physicians hear from administrators that they need to produce more. At the same time, they're being told by the variation-reduction team that they should do less. The reality is that the goal of most productivity initiatives is to increase the availability of physicians at times when physicians have traditionally not been available—weekends, evenings, in clinics, and so forth. This type of increase of physician productivity is not in conflict with variation reduction because we expect physicians to follow the variation-reduction standards during those extra or alternative time slots, too. Many physicians hear "increase productivity" as "do as much as you can for each patient," when it's actually aimed at increasing physician availability.

Several years ago, PAMF went through an initiative called Advanced Access, a series of tools and workshops where physicians and staff were trained to work more efficiently in the clinics so they could do more during each office visit. One concept taught was Max-Packing, the idea being that if a patient came in for a cold or some other acute problem, the physician would also use some of the visit time to check other matters: to see whether they had all their vaccinations, for example, or whether they needed to schedule a mammogram or some other kind of preventative health-maintenance issue.

Physicians ask, "Isn't variation reduction in direct conflict with the ideas of Advanced Access? You know, 'Do less, not more'?" We point out that what you're trying to do as a good variation-reduction physician is promote care that's appropriate, leaving out the unnecessary. A good example of this is the issue of how often a woman needs to have a Pap smear. It's now fairly well-established that yearly Pap smears are no longer necessary in most women. Every three years is now the accepted standard, so that adding a Pap smear to a visit for the acute problem is not something that you're likely to need to do. Not doing an unnecessary Pap smear opens up a slot to see another patient.

"WON'T THIS INTERFERE WITH MY AUTONOMY?"

Loss of autonomy is the fourth concern that physicians raise when thinking about variation reduction. For physicians, autonomy is a core issue. Training physicians takes a long time: four years of medical school and then three to five years (or more) of specialty training. All during this time the trainee physician is being told what to do. It's not surprising after this long apprenticeship that many physicians no longer want to take direction; they want to make decisions for themselves and they think the years of training have given them the right to do so. Now we come along as the variation-reduction team and start questioning their independent decisions.

Many physicians have an idealized vision of how medicine should be practiced. Television gave this vision a face: Marcus Welby, MD, the kindly General Practitioner who worked alone in a small office and was responsible only to himself and his patients. Dr. Welby could spend as much time as he needed during each visit; no group practice and no HMOs got between this doctor and his patients. The reality of practicing medicine today is, of course, much different. As reality takes physicians farther and farther away from the Dr. Welby ideal, physicians experience it as a loss of autonomy.

The solo practitioner is as close to the Dr. Welby ideal as one can get. When I first went into solo practice, I thought I could hang a "Closed" sign on the door any time I wanted to take time off. The reality was that I needed to be in a call group so that my patients would always have someone to turn to if I was not available—my first loss of autonomy but not the last.

When I eventually joined a group practice, my autonomy suffered again: now not only did I have to check with my call group when I wanted time off, I also had people looking over my shoulder making sure I was practicing medicine at a level the group thought was appropriate. When the group joined a larger medical organization, all of our physicians experienced another loss of autonomy. Now our collective fates were no longer directly in our hands but in the hands of an organization based 100 miles from where we practiced medicine.

These days, autonomy for physicians is pretty much an illusion. While some solo practitioners may still exist out in the hinterlands who depend on no one but themselves, the vast majority of physicians in the United States must always make compromises with the ideal of physician autonomy. For physicians working in a multi-specialty medical group, the loss of autonomy is counterbalanced by the benefits of working with a highly skilled team. The positives of working in a team range from the big issues, such as skill of the physician team members, to the more mundane, such as there is always someone to answer the phone even if your receptionist is out sick.

"ISN'T THIS JUST 'COOKBOOK MEDICINE'?"

A fifth concern is that standard-setting will reduce a physicians' practice to "cookbook medicine." What bothers physicians who use this term is that they worry that somehow the training they went through is no longer needed, that the treatment of the patient will be distilled down to a series of steps that anyone can follow. All those years of training and experience for nothing!

But does the use of a cookbook reduce the skill of an excellent cook or the nutrition provided by the food prepared by the recipe? I used to bristle at physicians' mention of cookbook medicine until I realized that cookbooks were exactly what I wanted to talk about. So the PAMF variation-reduction team took the metaphor and used it to our advantage. A good cook uses a cookbook. It's a starting point. You don't have to rigorously follow it; in fact, most good cooks vary a recipe depending on what is seasonally available and the people for whom they're cooking.

A standard is a recipe. It holds for about 80% to 90% of the patients that the physicians see, and the result of all the cooks in the kitchen following the same recipe is a consistent "dish" perfected with practice over time. But, just as a good cook changes a recipe as needed, a good physician matches a general standard of care to a specific patient. For some patients, the standard does not fit, and it would not be good clinical judgment to apply it.

Physicians have valid concerns regarding variation reduction, and the variation-reduction team listens avidly to those concerns. For the most part, we have been able to provide answers to the physicians' questions and win their engagement. That's crucial, because it's the engagement of physicians that powers not only the standard-setting process but its continued use.

CHAPTER 8

Growing Local Experts

When we first started the variation-reduction program at PAMF, we used the term "best practices" to refer to the standards we were developing. Some of the specialists rightly pointed out that since we were almost always dealing in areas where no evidence-based medicine existed, how did the variation-reduction team know that what we were doing was creating a "best" practice?

Ideally, physicians would like to have evidence-based medicine informing the vast majority of our clinical decision making; unfortunately, it's now estimated that 80% of physicians' daily activities haven't been subjected to evidence-based–medicine testing.[24] (This percentage is slightly better than the situation Jack Wennberg found in 1967, when only about 12% of Medicare expenditures could be attributed to evidence-based medicine.) But why is so little medicine evidence-based?

To be considered "evidence-based," a healthcare intervention must be validated in a randomized controlled trial (RCT). The Cochrane Collaboration (www.cochrane.org) has become the principal reviewer and repository of the findings of RCTs. In 2012, its library contained more than 5000 reviews of more than 100,000 RCTs, but even with this large number of reviews, it estimates that it needs to double the number of reviews just to cover the RCTs already done. Further, many current medical practices have never been subjected to an RCT. Many of the drugs we use are generic; because most drug RCTs are sponsored by the pharmaceutical industry, there is little or no funding to run RCTs on generic drugs.[25]

Typically, a physician faced with a clinical situation that has no evidence-based guidelines resorts to expert opinion. Also typically, the physician finds that experts have more than one opinion and that recommendations for care vary.

For example, in 2012, the U.S. Preventive Services Task Force recommended that physicians screen women from 21 to 65 for cervical cancer with Pap smears every three years and as infrequently as every five years for women 30 to 65 who have HPV testing done with the Pap test.[26] Initially, the American College of Obstetrics and Gynecology recommended continued yearly screening; in 2011 it changed its recommendations to every two years and after two normal paps every three years.[27]

So what does the physician do when seeing a 30-year-old woman? Pap tests every two years, three years, or five years? Physicians confronted with differing expert opinions frequently choose the more-aggressive or prevailing course of action. This tendency is not always to the patient's benefit. "Doing more" exposes patients to increased risk as well as increased cost. While the risk of an additional Pap smear is probably trivial, that's not the case with every test or intervention. For example, we now know that receiving an abdominal CT scan for suspected appendicitis increases a child's risk for childhood leukemia and brain tumor; emergency-room physicians can use abdominal ultrasound rather than the CT scan to avoid exposing children to radiation. However, a recent review of the use of CT scans in abdominal pain in children showed a dramatic increase in the use of CT scans, while the use of the safer ultrasound test has remained stable.[28] I recently was speaking to a group of Emergency Department (ED) physicians who were interested in examining variation in the ED. They raised the issue of the use of CT in children with abdominal pain: despite the increased risk of cancer, some surgeons will not see a child suspected of having appendicitis without a CT scan in hand.

Another example is hormone-replacement therapy (HRT). Twenty-plus years ago, it was standard practice for physicians to treat postmenopausal women with HRT. With long-term follow up, it was found that this practice placed the women at increased risk for certain types of cancers, so its routine use has, for the most part, been abandoned.

But don't physicians rely on clinical guidelines? Because a clinical-guideline process is required when a medical group signs an HMO-type contract, most medical organizations have many loose-leaf binders filled with health-plan—approved guidelines covering a wide variety of situations. These guidelines typically come from professional medical societies (both specialty and Primary Care) or from government agencies such as the U.S. Public Health Service. Typically, the organization has a guidelines committee that reviews the available medical literature on a yearly basis to see if current guidelines are still appropriate and revises them as necessary.

The committee also establishes new guidelines, choosing a topic, doing a literature search, reviewing the clinical evidence, and discussing the topic from a distance to answer the question, "What should one do, given a particular clinical situation?" The guidelines committee evaluates the strength of the evidence that is presented in the medical literature, tries to address all aspects of the clinical situation, and tries, for the most part, to adhere to national guidelines if such guidelines exist. But quite often, the physicians on a guidelines committee are not actually involved with taking care of the particular clinical entity under discussion, and so their recommendations carry little weight with practitioners.

A guidelines committee's final step is to spread a newly developed guideline throughout the organization, typically through a physician-education mechanism. Unfortunately, what happens most of the time is that the new guideline is sent out, disregarded, and forgotten. There is little follow up to see whether physicians are adhering to the guideline. The end result is one more binder on the shelf and—at best—inconsistent adherence to the guideline.

At the Palo Alto Medical Foundation, our physician leaders decided to freely admit that clinical decision making is often a question of expert opinion. Because most physicians' decisions are based on expert opinion anyway, we decided to rely on our own experts—that is, our specialists—to make decisions about common clinical situations. For our variation-reduction project, PAMF sidestepped broad clinical guidelines to focus on the root cause of local clinical variation; by doing so, we learned to value—and encourage—our own physicians' decisions to differ from national guidelines based on our own experience with our population of patients.

For example, well into our variation-reduction project, we received data from the Sutter Health Pharmacy Department showing extensive variation among PAMF Gastroenterologists in the treatment of chronic active hepatitis. Chronic active hepatitis is a blood-borne viral disease that not only creates chronic liver disease, but also increases the likelihood of the development of liver cancer. This is a very serious disease, and it is not something that can be easily treated. Further, the drugs that were and are being used to treat chronic active hepatitis are very expensive and have significant side effects, so physicians don't prescribe them lightly. Numerous medical journal articles have been published on who needs to be treated, and when, and how. The National Institutes of Health (NIH) convened a conference on this topic and established national guidelines for the treatment of this disease; the American College of Gastroenterology developed its own standards, which were similar, but not identical. (In retrospect, the fact that two very reputable organizations set two different standards said something about these standards themselves.)

The Sutter pharmacy staff drew my attention to the fact that PAMF Gastroenterologists weren't following *either* standard; instead, they were using large quantities of the expensive drugs to aggressively treat large numbers of their patients. In the interests of cost control, the pharmacy staff asked me to intervene. As the Managed Care Medical Director, I said I would look into it, but I was reluctant because doing so was contrary to our ethic of supporting physician groups as *they* select the clinical entities they work with in the variation-reduction process.

When I began to look at the data from the dozen PAMF Gastroenterologists, however, I soon realized that the varying practice wasn't attributable to all the Gastroenterologists; in fact, just two of them accounted for almost all of the variation. What's more, both Gastroenterologists had unusually large patient panels with chronic active hepatitis; in fact, they saw more patients with chronic active hepatitis than the rest of the PAMF Gastroenterologists combined.

So, practicing "management by walking around," I went and talked to these two physicians. Why did so many of their patients need to be treated so aggressively? Their reply was very interesting. They said that they knew that they were treating many more patients than the national guidelines would recommend, but their particular patient population was different than the national norm. In particular, they had a very high Asian population, and the Asian population was known in the gastroenterology literature to have increased risk—even above that of people already infected with the hepatitis virus—for developing liver cancer. It was their judgment that any abnormality in liver-function tests in an Asian patient was enough to start treatment for chronic active hepatitis.

Somewhat taken aback by their response, I said, "Well, you know this course of treatment is in direct contradiction to the NIH guidelines and your own specialty society guidelines as well." They said they knew that, but in good conscience, they couldn't *not* treat these patients, because they were at such high risk. Not yet having learned to rely on *our* expert opinion, I said to them, "This is really hubris for you two guys here in Palo Alto to go against national guidelines like this." They replied that they didn't care: they were seeing these patients, and the people who set up the national guidelines were not.

The two physicians really weren't being arrogant; they were just concerned for their patients. So I said to them, "Well, let's follow this along. We'll establish a registry and see how many patients *do* develop liver cancer." I thought it was going to be a very long-term project, and I wondered if we'd gain any really usable data. To my surprise, the issue of being out of step was settled about six months later, when the NIH came out with a revision of the guidelines which noted that Asians were a special, high-risk group for the development of liver cancer from chronic active hepatitis, and that they should be treated aggressively . . . basically what our two Gastroenterologists were already doing. To be honest, I'm not sure how we would have proceeded had the national standard not changed. I think we would have stuck with our method, gathered the data, then gotten all the GI physicians together to discuss the treatment standard. Eventually we would have reached our local consensus, even if it contradicted the national standard.

The lesson for me was not just that these two guys were ahead of their time; it was that it's important to really support the physicians who are seeing the patients. A committee sitting in another part of the country and trying to establish a national standard—however well-intentioned—can get it wrong. We know our patients best, and it's in everyone's best interest to let us establish best practices . . . and gather the evidence to back them up. PAMF is a large enough organization and sees enough patients that we have ample opportunities to collect the information we need to create local evidence-based medicine.

It was at about this time that the PAMF variation-reduction team decided to change the term "best practices" to "standard of care." At the Palo Alto Medical Foundation, we would deliver care that was based on a consensus of local specialists who know our patients the best and are aware of how our local populations might differ from the national norm.

CHAPTER 9

Understanding Variation

Before we could begin to reduce unwarranted variation, we needed to understand why variation exists in any form. Why do some physicians do more and others do less in the same clinical situation?

If physicians' main impetus is financial gain, as some critics charge and as seems in fact to be true in places like McAllen, Texas, you'd wonder why clinical variation occurs at all: why would any physician do less, rather than more? Certainly, the U.S. reimbursement system is set up to benefit physicians who perform procedures; physicians get paid relatively little for the cognitive work they do.

For example, over the last five years, PAMF's charge for a colonoscopy performed by a GI physician has been four times that of a consultation with that same physician. Both activities take about the same length of time, but the remuneration is far greater for the procedure than the consultation. It doesn't take long for new GI physicians to realize that their time is more lucratively spent doing the procedure than the consultation; some GI physicians no longer even see patients until they reach the endoscopy suite. This practice is now typical in most large groups. As an organization, PAMF has responded to the increased demand by patients for colonoscopy by hiring nurse practitioners to do the "colon talks." More patients screened equals more revenue generated.

So there's a structural incentive to do more and a structural disincentive to do less, let alone "nothing," like, say, spending time on patient education. Still, variation exists. Why?

The first major reason, I think, is a dichotomy between physicians' personality traits of activism and caution. Some physicians, like the two PAMF Gastroenterologists who aggressively treat chronic hepatitis, are activists. All physicians want to make their patients get better; activist physicians want to make it happen by doing something. It's easier to take action than to just sit and watch the patient. For activist physicians, *not* doing something is harder than doing something.

And of course, there is also a clear preference on the part of patients to have something done, particularly when they are referred—or self-refer—to a specialist. Often, the patients have already decided that they need a specific test based on what they have gleaned from the Internet or from family or friends or neighbors.

Often patients feel that if they go to the doctor's office and all the doctor does is talk to them, they really haven't gotten their money's worth. When I was a practicing Pulmonologist, I saw patients multiple times a year for their chronic lung problems. Typical office visits consisted of asking patients how they had been doing and what symptoms they were experiencing, then checking on whether they were taking their medications properly. We would spend most of the visit discussing how they were dealing with their chronic disabling illness and what strategies they could use to make life better.

Making sure that patients were following the regimen was clearly very important, but it was only during the fall visit, when they received an influenza vaccination, that patients really felt that they were getting something. It didn't matter that it was a rather routine injection; it was the physical act of doing something that made the patient feel that this visit was somehow better than the other visits during the year. Now I don't want to minimize the necessity of yearly flu vaccinations for patients at high risk for respiratory disease, but it would have been nice had the patients realized that their discussions with me on how to deal with this very difficult chronic disease were probably as important, if not more important, than receiving the vaccination.

Some physicians, on the other hand, are naturally cautious. When a new medication comes out, they're not willing to jump on the bandwagon no matter how hard-pressed by pharmaceutical representatives or tempted by advertising in the medical journals. They take a wait-and-see approach to new medications and new procedures, wanting to understand if the new thing is truly a safe and effective way of taking care of patients and to make sure that its risks don't outweigh the benefits received.

Not only are some physicians reluctant to use new medications, but there is at times federal regulatory reluctance to approve new drugs. The classic example is the drug thalidomide, which was widely used in Europe as a sleep aid and to treat morning sickness of pregnancy. The FDA was reluctant to approve this drug, especially in pregnant women—a level of caution that was proven to be correct when it was recognized that the drug was causing children to be born with severe defects to their limbs.[29]

The second major reason for variation is physicians' training. When my team has spoken with physicians who have a pattern of higher utilization, and asked them why their practice pattern differs, the first answer that comes up—not surprisingly—is, "This is the way I was trained." I remember looking at Urology data and noticing that one—and only one—of the Urologists was doing an ultrasound whenever he saw a patient with infertility. When I asked why, he said, "Because that's the way I was trained—isn't everyone doing it?" When I said that he was the only one doing this test for this condition, he said, "So I'll stop." And he did—lowering the cost to the patient without lowering quality of care.

Also unsurprisingly, "This is the way I was trained" is the answer we get when we talk to physicians who don't do as much as their colleagues. One of the most worrisome things patients can hear from their doctors is that they have a "spot on the lung." This phrase raises the specter of lung cancer, a terrible disease with a poor prognosis even in the face of modern treatment. The term Pulmonologists use for "spot on the lung" is "pulmonary nodule." Evaluation of pulmonary nodules has changed with the advent of several newer technologies: the CT scan and fiber-optic bronchoscopy. Now, with the guidance of the CT scan, biopsies of the lung can be made more safely, avoiding the need for a major operation to remove a pulmonary nodule and the surrounding lung tissue. The Pulmonologists were interested in examining variation in the way they evaluate pulmonary nodules. The variation-reduction team found the typical two- to three-fold variation seen in most clinical situations. When we looked at the reasons for the variation, we found that Pulmonologists with the higher average cost per patient were using these new techniques while their lower-cost colleagues were not. Additional investigation revealed that the patients seen by the low-cost Pulmonologists had a higher frequency of undergoing surgery for lung biopsy. When we asked those Pulmonologists why they weren't using the less-invasive bronchoscopy biopsy, we heard the usual refrain, "That's the way I was trained." So training can be the cause of inappropriate under-utilization as well as over-utilization.

Temperament and training have a massive impact on variation in physicians' practice patterns, especially for physicians who practice independently. Interestingly, that impact appears to be attenuated in specialties that typically practice in teams.

As a Pulmonologist myself, I've had a lot of experience working with teams. When I was practicing, all the Pulmonologists in our group met every morning to go over the patients who were in the critical-care unit. We showed each other the X-rays and we told each other our plans for our patients over the next 24 hours. There was a practical reason for doing this: no Pulmonologist could be on call 24 hours a day, seven days a week, and each of us needed to be able to sign out a patient to a colleague who would need to understand what was going on with the patient.

Each day's meeting included an active discussion among the Pulmonologists about the care plan that the primary Pulmonologist was creating for that patient. Over time, the practice patterns of the various Pulmonologists—even though we had different points of view and had been trained at different institutions—seemed to merge into a common way of taking care of patients. In retrospect, what our Pulmonology group was doing was creating an informal local standard, one of the key elements in the variation-reduction methodology.

Apart from isolated examples of physicians mostly interested in the economics of healthcare, the sources of unwarranted clinical variation throughout our healthcare system are understandable and honest. Nothing is gained by accusatory or antagonist attempts to change physicians' behavior by administrative fiat. By showing our colleagues the data about variation, querying them about their practices, and engaging their interest in the variation we find, the variation-reduction team is able to clearly separate warranted variation from unwarranted variation and simply concentrate on helping to reduce the latter.

CHAPTER 10

Pillars of Variation Reduction

W hen Dr. Trujillo, Dr. Knapp, and I formed PAMF's variation-reduction steering committee, we realized that we didn't really have a standard way of thinking about the process we were undertaking. Our ultimate goal was to create a variation-reduction process that was physician-owned and operated, but to get there we would have to engage our colleagues and scale up.

We decided that we needed a set of principles that we could easily state. We came up with what we called the Five Pillars of Variation Reduction: affordability, expert knowledge, physician engagement, resources, and useful data. We used these pillars as the organizing principle of innumerable presentations we made to physicians and administrators to win them over to the variation-reduction cause. (Later, we added "value" as the foundation for it all.) Figure 4 shows the slide we created using pillars from the Greek Temple of Asclepius, god of medicine.

AFFORDABILITY IS THE ANSWER

The first pillar of our project is that affordability is mission-critical for the Palo Alto Medical Foundation.

PAMF has long-standing experience in the HMO business: currently about 22% of our patients are insured by HMOs; 10 years ago this number was 45%. (The decline in patients with HMO insurance was caused by the rise of high-deductible health plans. Using these types of insurance plans, employers could shift part of the cost of healthcare to the employee. This made premiums for the high-deductible plans less than premiums for the

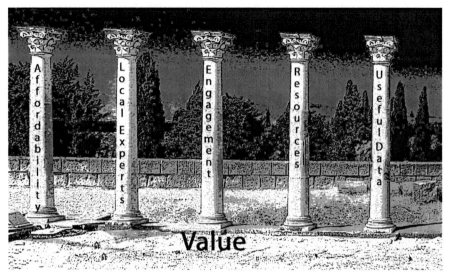

FIGURE 4. Temple of Asclepius, Pillars of Hippocrates. Illustration based on a photo by Torsten Huckert.

HMOs.) We have been taking care of pre-paid patients with HMO insurance since the early 1970s and have been very successful in doing this type of medical care. Our physicians are well-versed in providing appropriate care for the patients with HMO insurance, trying to do as much of the care within the organization as possible.

Our assumption in the past had been that patients with PPO insurance used more care than patients with HMO insurance for two reasons. First, patients with HMO insurance were subjected to a pre-authorization gatekeeping process; second, treatment of patients with HMO insurance was based on the HMO's identification of what groups of patients need, not on what the individual patient wants. Patients with PPO insurance didn't have either of these restrictions, so if one physician was unwilling to provide a service a patient wanted, the patient could just go to another physician who would.

In recent years, however, we had become concerned by evidence that suggested that PAMF physicians were doing more for our patients with HMO insurance than for a like group of patients on the fee-for-service model. After analyzing the issue, I confirmed that this new situation *was*, in fact, occurring. Three explanations could account for the change. First, there was anecdotal evidence that the constraint in service was the physician's decision: when I would talk to the physicians, they would say things like, "Well, I know that patients in HMOs don't have out-of-pocket expenses for this test, so I'm likely to order it for them. But the patients on the fee-for-service plans, I sort of think twice about it, because I know that they have high deductibles." That was an unusual response at first, but it became commonplace as high-deductible plans became more and more prevalent.

A second potential explanation was competition: physicians were ordering the care, and patients on fee-for-service plans wanted to get the care, but they felt that our prices were too high, so they would, for example, go down the street to a freestanding imaging center where they could get an MRI done for a much lower cost than we could provide. We didn't see these outside reports coming in, though, so I couldn't confirm that patients were going down the street to a cheaper vendor.

All I could document statistically was the third reason, that patients considered cost an all-or-nothing issue: patients who had the high-deductible fee-for-service plans were just saying, "No. I can't afford to do that, and I'm not going to have that procedure or imaging study."

As it became clear that the market for healthcare was changing, and that the large payers in our area were shifting from traditional insurance plans to the self-funded type plans, it also became clear that patients were engaging in self-rationing, without and even against the advice of their physicians. To keep providing high-quality care for our patients, we needed to take proactive steps to make healthcare more affordable.

"YOU'RE THE EXPERTS"

The second pillar of variation reduction is that the physicians are the experts. Although the variation-reduction team may have initiated the conversation about variation reduction and educated physicians about the variation-reduction process, the physicians themselves are the ones who successfully complete any project.

"You're the experts; we're not," we tell our colleagues time and again. While this may seem to be an obvious statement, in fact, it is the basis of one of our major strategies, which is key to engaging practitioners in variation reduction. The strategy is called the "one-down" approach; it is best summarized as a way to encourage physicians to understand—and believe—that they have the dominant, authoritative, and controlling role in the variation-reduction process.[30]

Some would say that attributing dominance, authority, and control to physicians shouldn't be a difficult task, but remember we are bringing physicians together to discuss their performance, and they often come to initial variation-reduction meetings suspicious, hostile, and defensive. "Just tell us what you want us to do," they sometimes say, impatiently, their body language screaming "We've been here before." And with good reason: the typical paradigm for institutional change is leadership deciding what needs to change and by how much. Physicians are brought into the process only to learn in what way they are outliers to the new one true way and to learn how they are to effect the required change; whether leadership's underlying premise is correct is not up for discussion.

I remember a meeting I sat in on 10 years ago between PAMF Oncologists and the medical director of one of our large HMO health plans. PAMF's Oncologists are well-respected by their colleagues; as a department, they have the highest patient satisfaction of all the specialty departments. It's a strong department with a lot of strong personalities. This medical director demanded the Oncologists use plan-approved chemotherapy regimens and report their patients' progress to the health plan's nurse case managers. He told them that whether or not they agreed, the nurse case managers would be calling the patients directly to ask if their doctors were following the health plan–approved regimen. I was astounded by the performance, but unsurprised that the Oncologists basically decided to ignore his dictum; the initiative died quietly.

Any physician would bristle at such an approach, and the variation-reduction team was determined not to go down that path. Before we ask to meet with a group of physicians, we do our research, we accumulate interesting data about the physicians' variation, and we invariably generate our own ideas about projects this group of physicians could undertake. So we could take the one-up approach and tell the physicians what to do. But we know that if the physicians don't select their own projects, there will be no engagement. And without engagement, there will be no commitment to change. So we place ourselves in the one-down position from the very beginning. For example, when we ask to meet with a group of physicians, all we do is describe the need for PAMF to become more affordable and increase value to our patients, introduce the variation-reduction process, say that leadership is committed to it as a general principle, give a couple of examples of the process in action, then leave the what, the how, and the how much up to the physicians.

(A few years ago, I was teaching a group of Sutter Health medical directors about how we use the one-down approach. After the class, a woman medical director came up to me and told me that while she had not previously heard the term "one down," she was well-versed in its technique because she had been using it most of her life in dealing with men!)

Because initial variation-reduction meetings have a certain amount of tension in them, we try to dispel that tension by changing the dynamic in the room. Most physicians, whether they want to admit it or not, are intimidated by having their practices reviewed, even if they feel that they're doing an above-average job—and, of course, everybody feels that they're doing an above-average job. This sense of dread in being reviewed is muscle memory: physicians are frequently reviewed by their mentors during training, and most of us have strong memories of an unpleasant experience with a review process that didn't go well. Physicians who think that the variation-reduction process is just another one of these exercises that will point out their flaws are unlikely to engage. By focusing on physicians' status as experts, we are trying to distance ourselves from that approach.

So when the variation-reduction team met with the Oncology Department, we were determined not to repeat their history with previous cost-reduction efforts. Before the meeting, the Oncologists had heard about the variation-reduction process from other specialty groups that were already involved, and they had decided among themselves that they would like to examine variation in the way they treated breast cancer. They made that known, so before the initial meeting, the variation-reduction team prepared a data set for the 800 new breast cancer cases seen by the Oncologists over the last four years. We broke out the charges by Oncologists in four categories: office visits, lab, imaging, and medication, which we divided into the four major breast cancer drugs: neulasta/neupogen, taxotere, Herceptin, and Taxol.

One of the main techniques of the one-down approach is to ask simple questions. After we present data to the physicians showing variation, the first simple question that we always ask is, "Why do you think this variation exists?" So I showed the Oncologists their variation graph and asked the question, "We don't understand why there is so much variation; do you have any ideas?" They looked at the data with laser-like focus, then immediately said the variation we'd found was due to the fact that we had grouped all the patients with breast cancer together; had we had separated the patients by stages of cancer, they said, most of the variation would be eliminated. Using the one-down approach, I thanked them for the insight and said, "We'll re-do our queries to separate out the stages and get back to you." My immediate acquiescence to their request gave them the sense that they had control of the situation and increased their engagement in the process.

In the meantime, I asked, would the Oncologists be willing to look at the data we had? They were, and they saw that the variation was, for the most part, in their use of the drugs. Of the four drugs we'd charted, Herceptin was high on the list as to cost, but the Oncologists told us that they prescribed it only if a patient met specific pathology criteria, so we shouldn't bother to look at it for variation. Again we immediately agreed, and moved on. The costly white-cell stimulator drugs, however, showed significant variation. Here the Oncologists paused; while they still wanted the data broken down by the stage of the cancer, they were more than willing to begin looking at their use of these drugs. Had we not used the one-down approach, had we not agreed with their concerns, had we required them to look at the white-cell stimulators, I'm sure the conversation would have been contentious.

Getting data on the patients' stage of breast cancer turned out to be a huge project, requiring the variation-reduction team to perform a manual audit of the 800 patient records. (Subsequently, we developed the ability to do text searches of our electronic medical records, which provides the patient's stage in up to 80% of the cases.) We re-analyzed the data and saw the same variation. When we went back to the Oncologists, they were surprised that the variation persisted, but in the face of this new evidence, they were willing to acknowledge that they weren't all treating their patients with breast cancer in the same way and that they needed to create a standard to follow.

It's important to get to a place where the physicians are willing to accept the data. After that, if the simple question "Why do you think this variation exists?" gets the conversation started, then our job is pretty easy. More often than not, however, the question is met with a blank stare or an "I don't know. It really puzzles me." At this point, we ask a basic clinical question. For example, with a Urologist we might ask, "What do you do when you see a patient with a kidney stone?" Sometimes the answer is brief and general; in that case, a member of the variation-reduction team prompts a more specific response by saying, "Tell me exactly what you do first, and then, after that, what you do next."

The technique is to try to get the physician into "teacher mode." Physicians in general like to teach, and, in particular, like to teach other physicians. If you can get them to very clearly state what their thought process is when they're seeing the patient, then you can get other physicians in the room to engage.

The typical response when you get this kind of conversation going is, "Well, when I see this kind of patient, I do this."

And then another specialist in the room will say, "Wait a minute! I don't do that unless the following circumstances occur."

That's the discussion that you really want to begin, because it teases out the decision-making process that physicians go through for these common clinical situations. Holding this type of discussion is one of the building blocks for the development of the standard of care that the specialists are going to create. The skillful variation-reduction facilitator helps physicians be very clear about their thought processes in deciding to order a test or do surgery. Those are the key pieces of information that we need to articulate so that others can constructively respond.

"THEY'RE THE EXPERTS, STUPID"

Our third pillar of variation reduction is the concept that the variation-reduction team doesn't have the answers and that success requires everyone's engagement. This third principle is actually a restatement of the second one, and it's an example of the tactic of "tell 'em, then tell 'em again" so that they (and we) will remember. The fact that the physicians are the experts is so important that it requires emphasis to make sure that everybody understands that this process is different from any other process that physicians have gone through in the past when reviewing their own practices.

The variation-reduction team doesn't have the answers; we are not coming in with preconceived notions on what the standards should be and how they should be developed. When speaking to our colleagues, we take care to avoid using terms like "over-utilizers" and "under-utilizers" (let alone "good" and "bad" doctors). We don't even use terms like "outliers." We just present the variation-reduction data and say, "We don't understand why there's variation here."

While our variation-reduction team has become well-versed in the one-down technique, it's not uncommon for some of the physicians at initial meetings to take the one-up bit in their mouths and start accusing each other of being bad doctors. I recall meeting with the Sports Medicine physicians on knee arthroscopy. One of the physicians started down the bad doctor path. It was "clear" to him, he said, that surgeons who did fewer procedures (especially the ones who did fewer procedures than he did) were not doing a good job and, in fact, why was the group "letting these surgeons operate" at all?

We pulled him back before we all went over that cliff by reminding everyone of our basic tenet—that warranted variation does exist—and pointing out that we had not yet uncovered whether the variation we were looking at was warranted or unwarranted. By sticking to the one-down approach, which tells us not to label "good" practice and "bad" practice, we model a respectful behavior and a nonjudgmental approach to the data. We believe that the words we use and the behaviors we model subtly influence the physicians in the meeting to do the same. Had we allowed the surgeon to label some of his colleagues as "bad," he might well worry that in a future meeting he might receive the same label and might not want to participate.

"WE CAN GET YOU THAT INFORMATION"

Our fourth pillar of variation reduction is that the purpose of the variation-reduction team is to be the physicians' resource for improving quality and becoming more affordable. We encourage physicians who participate in the program to bring us clinical issues that have bothered them and for which they'd like to have data. A number of specialists have asked us to gather information on the use of medications in certain clinical situations. For example, anemia is a common consequence of chronic kidney disease, and the nephrologists were interested in their collective use of erythropoietin (the drug that stimulates red blood cell production). They wanted to see data on the way they were ordering this drug. Using pharmacy data, we were able to answer the clinical question that the doctors were asking: "Is there a difference in the way we are using this medication to treat patients with this condition?"

The ability to answer clinical questions that physicians raise gives the variation-reduction project credibility. Even if the information gathered didn't have a direct effect on the affordability of care at PAMF, it's a very useful technique in getting physicians engaged in the process. But, in fact, the ability to gather and analyze evidence to answer questions in clinical practice is crucial to variation reduction, so much so that we're working toward a future in which providing physicians with data is our main and perhaps only role. As we assist the specialties to organize themselves into variation-reduction teams, this work will become part of the standard work of all physicians at PAMF. It has to: PAMF has 25 specialty Departments; when we add in the Primary Care Departments and special-interest groups such as weight management, we have 30 different areas. Currently PAMF has five physicians working part time on the variation-reduction project; six specialties with multiple projects per area can quickly overwhelm even the most enthusiastic team member. And we know that no matter how many physicians we add to the team, the demand will always be greater than the number of team members we have. So the physician groups must take on this task themselves.

At PAMF, the variation-reduction team is currently developing a front end for our data warehouse. Any physician will be able to go to the front end, enter a few query terms such as specialty, diagnosis, and/or procedure, and see data on a specific clinical variation at PAMF. If the raw data piques the physician's interest, the variation-reduction team will provide more detailed information, but the initiating physician will be responsible for setting up the meetings, showing the data, facilitating the discussions, and seeing that a standard is set. The variation-reduction team will feed back to these self-motivated physicians the effect of their standards.

"WE DIDN'T SAY IT WAS PERFECT"

Our fifth pillar of variation reduction is, from an operational point of view, perhaps the most important: it states that the variation-reduction team commits generally to producing useful data—which may not necessarily describe the particular data set that we're presenting to physicians at this moment in time. We acknowledge right from the beginning that any given data set may not be perfect.

In fact, we don't even look for perfect data sets. We look for good data sets that get the discussion going. Data is necessary to the process, but are not sufficient. It is the engagement of the physicians, rather than developing a perfect data set, that's the goal of the variation-reduction project staff. Stating up front that we don't believe that our data are perfect decreases the number of defensive arguments that physicians give us about the data.

At the beginning of our project, a typical conversation about data with physicians began with someone pointing out the one obvious error that we missed, then saying, "Well, if this one error is there, the whole data set is probably wrong, so we're going to discount the entire project." That was a conversation stopper, and that's what we don't want to happen. Over time we learned to acknowledge up front that we knew we had problems with the data, and we were able to begin dialogues with, "Here's what we have so far. Can you tell us how to fix the data set so we can make this usable for you?"

What we have found after dealing with many different specialties is that the pattern is always the same. The physicians look at the data and say, "Well, here are the obvious mistakes, and we're sure that if you just correct these mistakes the variation will disappear." So we go back and change our queries to meet their objections, rerun the data, and lo and behold, the variation persists. Typically, it takes one or two or three rounds of refining the queries for the physicians to be convinced that the variation in the data is due not to some anomaly of the data-gathering process, but to the practices of the individual physicians regarding this particular clinical entity.

This strategy of freely admitting that the data is not perfect, and that we're not striving for perfect data sets, is another example of the one-down approach discussed as part of the second pillar of variation reduction. What's interesting about this particular concept isn't that physicians have some difficulty accepting the idea that we're looking only for good, not perfect, data. It's that the people who really have a problem with it are the information technology folks. The IT Department is in the business of creating perfect data. Typically, the data that they produce is claims data that go to the insurance companies. You certainly do want to have error-free submissions to the insurance companies; you also want to make sure that your books balance at the end of the month. So the IT Department has the mindset that its data have to be completely accurate, and they had a lot of trouble with our request to just get the raw data and not worry about it being perfect: if we don't have every single case, it really doesn't matter, because when we're looking at hundreds of cases per doctor, missing one or two is not going to make that much of a difference in the overall variation.

That's not to say that we're not careful with our queries. Missing an occasional patient is not much of a problem, but missing whole sections of data is; it could imply variation that isn't present or miss variation that is. A good data set gets the discussion started, while a bad data set just brings up data-problem issues rather than the clinical issues.

Our biggest learning curve in our dealings with the IT department was that it will give you exactly what you ask for—nothing more, nothing less. As in the classic computer adage, garbage in equals garbage out, and we learned to be very careful about making sure that the queries we ask of the data warehouse are exactly right to get the output we need.

THE FOUNDATION

Initially, we didn't use the term "value" when we were distilling our variation-reduction principles into the five pillars. As our project evolved, however, we began to realize that value was the foundation on which everything else depended. Value is a combination of appropriateness of care, quality of care, and affordability.

Previous efforts by PAMF leadership had stressed affordability only when speaking to physicians, a discussion that made the physicians uncomfortable. Physicians don't like to talk about affordability because they don't want to feel that their medical judgment is influenced by the cost of the treatment, or conflate the cost of care with the care of the patient. Physicians would prefer to work in a world where the cost of care is irrelevant. Unfortunately that world never existed and certainly is not the world we live in today.

In the past, physicians always wanted to shift the conversation from affordability to quality of care: it's easy for physicians to talk about quality, because everyone wants to provide the highest-quality service for their patients. By introducing appropriateness into the equation, we were able to add an important issue that variation reduction specifically raises: value to the patient. Shifting the conversation from cost to value makes the conversation easier for the variation-reduction team when we talk with physicians. It also serves as a model for the conversations that physicians will need to have with their patients: when physicians decide as a group to create and follow a standard of care, they need to explain the new regime to their patients. (Imagine patients' reactions when told by their physicians that they are not going to receive a procedure "because of the cost." The patients could easily misinterpret the decision to mean that it's too bad they're not rich or had better insurance so that this valuable procedure could be done. No one would want to have that discussion!) Physicians should discuss care with patients in terms of its value to them as an individual: "Will this procedure be of value to you?"

♦ ♦ ♦

Part II concentrated on the changing environment for healthcare in the United States and the changes physicians need to make in our thinking and our practice. The first task of PAMF's variation-reduction team was to help our physicians understand that healthcare in the United States is rapidly changing both nationally and locally. At the beginning of the project, it was especially difficult for some of our colleagues to accept that change was occurring, since they personally had yet to feel any effect on their practices or their income. As the changes brought on by the Affordable Care Act begin to take effect, some physicians want to wait until the transformation of the healthcare system changes the way physicians are paid. But it's getting harder and harder to wait. Change is here, now, and with it come challenges.

So our second task was to decide how we were going to change our practices to meet these challenges. PAMF chooses to embrace change by providing increased value to our patients. As an organization, we have committed to the concept that the changes we need to make are for all our patients, regardless of their type of insurance: HMO, Accountable Care Organization (ACO), or fee-for-service. Every patient will receive services (such as help from nurse case managers and social workers) that in the past had been limited to patients with HMO insurance. We are setting local standards to reduce unwarranted variation and decrease unnecessary and inappropriate care so that we can increase value for all.

Part III:

Variation Reduction by the Book

CHAPTER 11

Is Variation Reduction Right for You?

I f you've made it to this section of the book, you're probably interested in creating your own variation-reduction program. Who are you? Perhaps you're a medical group's board member. Perhaps you work in managed care. Perhaps you're part of the physician leadership of a specialty group. Whoever you are, for variation reduction to take hold, you'll need to work with physicians as peers to foster a new paradigm for change.

If the physicians in your setting perceive your variation-reduction project as just another managed care–type attempt to reduce utilization from the top down, this process will fail. In fact, quite a few common and otherwise reasonable practices will cause the process to fail. So I thought I'd pass along some tips on how you can avoid critical mistakes as you set up a variation-reduction project of your own.

Personally, I'm not much of a DIY-type guy. I typically plunge into a project only to realize that I don't have the right tools or the parts I'll need to get the job done. Everything takes longer than I predict, and I spend a good part of my time and effort recovering from mistakes. In retrospect, that's what I did with my initial variation-reduction project at PAMF. Faced with the Aetna challenge, I plunged head first into trying to deal with the issue and learned as I went along; I was two years into the process before I really knew what I was doing. It was probably only because of my long-held position as Managed Care Medical Director that I was given so much time to flail (and fail), eventually leading to the transformation of my quixotic project into an institutionally sponsored program with dedicated staff, budget, support from leadership, and incontrovertible results.

PAMF began this project nine years ago, when the healthcare climate was not as turbulent as it is now and the penalties for failure were less extreme. If you have the time and the inclination, then using a trial-and-error approach may work for you, too. Unfortunately, healthcare reform and market changes are forcing physicians and medical groups to change more quickly than ever before. Maybe one shot is all you'll get at this kind of experimentation, so I'd like to help you learn from our experience at PAMF.

I like cookbooks. I like cookbooks when I try to cook and I like cookbooks in medicine. So what follows here is, in effect, the PAMF cookbook for variation reduction. Feel free to change the recipe to use local ingredients and season to your own taste. But before you start, check that your kitchen has the equipment you'll need for your project and that your fellow cooks are ready, able, and enthusiastic. Do you have what it takes to start a variation-reduction project? At a minimum, make sure you have robust data, a workable group structure, organizational commitment, and physician engagement.

ROBUST DATA

This first issue is a deal breaker. Are you able to collect, access, organize, and analyze the data that will show variation? Until recently, I had assumed that all medical groups had this type of information because this is the information needed to bill Medicare, Medicaid, and any commercial insurance plan.

However, when one of our local safety-net hospitals asked me to consult on how it could develop a variation-reduction project, I learned that it doesn't bill any insurance company. It's funded by state and local agencies and submits no bills to any type of insurance plan. Because its physicians do not bill for their services, it has no central repository of what work is done. We were able to find some small amount of data for them to work with, based on referral and ordering patterns, but nothing robust.

Aside from this rather small population of physician groups that see patients who seek safety-net care, I believe that most medical groups have the wherewithal to generate the encounter data they need for variation reduction. When I started my solo practice in pulmonary we had paper "superbills" and a pegboard ledger system. Those days are long gone. Most medical groups of any size bill with an electronic system, especially since Medicare requires that submissions be sent electronically. All electronic billing systems include the data needed for variation reduction: patient identifier, identifier for the physician who performed the service, and date of service. In addition, all electronic billing systems track procedure codes, which describe *what* was done, and diagnosis codes, which describe *why* it was done.

(Most billing systems use Current Procedural Terminology [or CPT] codes to classify procedures. CPT codes can have modifiers that identify specifics about the procedure, for example, modifiers that name assistant surgeons or indicate that a second procedure was performed at the same time as the principal procedure. Most billing systems use ICD-9 codes to classify diagnoses. Typically billing systems have four to eight locations for ICD-9 code entry. Each diagnosis must pertain to the procedure. So, for example, an Orthopedist who sees a new patient with a broken hip who also has degenerative osteoarthritis would enter both ICD-9 codes.)

You'll need data that's downloaded into a data warehouse on a regular basis; PAMF does this every day. In addition, you'll need to have some way to get the information out of the data warehouse and into usable form. Many software packages can extract data; some billing systems may be able to give you this type of report directly. The first stop for anyone interested in starting a variation-reduction program is a trip to your business office to talk with that department's IT guru. That person will be able to help you learn the capabilities of your system and whether you'll need a separate data warehouse for your work.

A WORKABLE GROUP STRUCTURE

Can any group of physicians initiate a variation-reduction project? Or is variation reduction the province only of the large, multi-specialty medical group?

Clearly, a large, multi-specialty medical group, with most or all of the specialties covered by salaried physicians, is an ideal organizational structure to undertake variation reduction. But as we've learned, you don't need an ideal organizational structure to do variation reduction. What you need is the group's willingness to participate in the effort. If the group acknowledges that physicians play a role in driving the cost of healthcare, and that as a profession we have a responsibility to our individual patients, as well as our community, then any group of physicians can begin.

As our team helped spread variation reduction throughout the Sutter Health system, we encountered many other types of physician organizations, ranging from much-smaller medical groups with limited internal specialists to medical groups that were purely Primary Care, to medical groups that were independent-practice associations (IPAs). Each type of physician group practice poses a different set of problems.

The typical issue for the smaller multi-specialty medical group is that it may have only one or two physicians in any specialty. It's hard to recognize variation when you have only one or two points of data. To get around this issue, a smaller medical group needs to be willing to share its data with other groups, a practice that creates its own difficulties. It's one thing for PAMF specialists to sit down with their partners and discuss clinical variation. In the beginning we didn't all know one another but we were willing to do it because we were all stakeholders in the same group. It's a different dynamic when two different groups sit down to discuss variation, especially when the physicians have never met before. It's not impossible, but it's difficult.

Specialty variation is the most fiscally rewarding initial vehicle for variation reduction. For a medical group comprised of only Primary Care physicians, specialty variation is a very difficult topic to discuss. Because the specialists are contracted for the patients with HMO insurance, the group typically worries that the discussion could offend the specialists to the point that they would no longer contract with the group. For Primary Care–only medical groups, it's probably better to deal with variation within Primary Care rather than starting with variation in specialty care.

IPAs pose the greatest challenge, because they are formed, for the most part, to deal only with the managed care/HMO-type business. IPA members are independent physicians who have agreed to contract together for HMO business. Members most often practice in their own small offices, with their own medical records. Each IPA is different. Some are tightly bound together and use identical billing systems; others prize their independence, leaving each member to practice as it sees fit. A common model is to pay Primary Care physicians not by service, but per patient per month. Specialists are paid fee-for-service.

IPAs leave non-HMO business up to the individual physicians, who bill Medicare or a commercial insurance company directly. So the IPA has information on physicians only with regard to patients with HMO insurance. This brings us back to PAMF's original problem with Aetna's project, which gathered too little data. For PAMF, patients with HMO insurance represented much less than half, and sometimes less than a quarter, of all patients seen by a given physician; when we started looking at individual clinical entities, the number got even smaller. The smaller the number of patients, the less powerful the data.

What makes dealing with IPAs even more difficult is that physicians frequently belong to more than one IPA. In dealing with the Sutter IPA in Sacramento, for example, we found that specialists, in particular, frequently belong not only to the Sutter IPA, but to competing IPAs. While leadership of the Sutter IPA was interested in doing variation reduction, they had considerable second thoughts when they realized that although the Sutter IPA alone would be spending money to generate data, develop standards, and implement those standards, some of the benefit of its work would go to competing IPAs because it was not realistic to expect the specialist to use the standard Sutter developed only on patients of the Sutter IPA.

When I discussed this issue with the Sutter IPA leadership, they told me that one of the solutions that they had thought of was to make participation in the Sutter IPA exclusive; that is, any physician who was a member of the Sutter IPA could not be a member of any other IPA. While the Sutter IPA leadership thought that this was a reasonable solution, the leadership of its parent organization, Sutter Health, did not think that this was a good idea at all: they wanted all physicians in the Sacramento area to feel that they were part of the Sutter system because they wanted these physicians to use the Sutter hospitals. To exclude any physician was anathema to the Sutter Health leadership. Competing forces such as these are obviously real and need to be recognized.

If a group of physicians were to ask me how they should organize to take on the task of improving the value of healthcare through variation reduction, I would advise them to organize themselves into a medical group. The most significant advantage of the medical group structure for a variation-reduction project is that there's no obstacle to sharing information within the group. In the IPA setting, information sharing is limited to those situations where the members of the IPA have agreed to participate in an HMO plan. (IPAs cannot contract for the PPO business because regulators have deemed the practice to be anti-competitive and a potential anti-trust violation.)

A second advantage of the medical group structure when attempting variation reduction is the ability to share the cost of information systems. It's expensive for solo or small medical practices to purchase the needed electronic billing and medical record systems because of the large capital investment required. Because medical groups are investing for many more physicians, they typically have the resources to make these purchases.

A third reason is that physicians who agree to join a group have already made the leap to work together, so agreeing to standards and reducing variation comes easier. Physicians in IPAs cherish their independence so it's more of a struggle to get them to work in a standard manner.

ORGANIZATIONAL COMMITMENT

Organizational commitment is essential for the success of a variation-reduction project. Why would an organization commit to this kind of project? It may be that becoming more affordable is part of an organization's mission to provide higher value care, or there may be a sense that the organization needs to take a stand against its ever-rising cost. It may be just enlightened self-interest.

Whatever the reason, the organization has to take the long view to get to its goal. It's unlikely that things will change in 3 months or even 6 months. Most variation-reduction projects take 6 to 12 months before the team can even start to think about seeing whether a standard has had any effect. And even then, the effect may not be measurable as monetary return on investment (ROI).

In discussions with physician leaders, I've mentioned that variation-reduction projects could have a monetary ROI of zero; in fact, ROI could actually be negative. The physicians were somewhat surprised that anyone would want to think about an initiative with a negative ROI. I asked them, "Are you losing market share? Are you being eliminated from narrow networks?

Are your patients complaining that they can't afford the care that you're recommending? If you answer any of those questions 'yes,' then I'd suggest that ROI is not the only way to look at a variation-reduction project."

Organizational commitment to variation reduction means committing resources to the project. Trying to create transformational change on a shoestring, or as a part-time process, is less likely to succeed. Although PAMF did head down the variation-reduction path with only one physician (me) and no data-analytic support, this type of start lessens the likelihood of an early success. It took PAMF a while, but as we achieved each success, the organization committed more and more resources to the process. (I knew that I had organizational commitment when I got a budget for food for the doctors' meetings!)

What should you ask of your organization if you are considering undertaking variation reduction? I would start with three types of resources: a physician champion (see the next section of this chapter), a data analyst, and an administrative assistant. All three resources are vital to the success of variation reduction. For each individual you bring on board, you'll measure start-up costs not so much in money, but in time. It will take a new physician champion time to learn how to use data and how to lead discussion groups; later that time is reduced. Likewise it will take a new data analyst time to set up or learn procedures for accessing and organizing the data; after that, the data analyst's time can be reduced. In addition, it will take time for the physician champion and the data analyst to learn to work in partnership to develop the necessary data sets. Collaboration is the key: typically the physician knows the medical aspect of the data but not how to get the data and organize it; just as typically, the data analyst knows how to get the data and organize it but doesn't grasp its medical significance. And unless PAMF is different from any other medical group, scheduling physician meetings is not a trivial task; it will take time for a new administrative assistant to develop the skills and persistence necessary to organize physicians and persuade them to attend meetings.

How much time each resource spends on variation reduction over the long run is determined by how large the organization is, as well as how committed to the process it is. A good start in a medium-sized medical group is between 0.25 and 0.5 FTE for the physician champion and data analyst and 0.25 FTE for the administrative assistant. As the project gets rolling, you'll need more personnel. Currently PAMF has a total of 4.25 FTEs on the variation-reduction team (2.0 FTE physician champions, 1.5 FTE analysts, 0.5 FTE program director, and 0.25 FTE administrative assistant). This number doesn't count the specialist physicians who meet to decide on the standards. PAMF pays the physicians for this committee work just as we pay for other committee work that the foundation decides is necessary for the good of the whole organization.

In addition to resources, an organization must commit its leadership. When the organization's leadership talks to physicians about how they intend to solve the affordability problem, they need to mention variation reduction at every opportunity. It's not enough for just the variation-reduction leadership to talk about the process and the successes; rank-and-file physicians need to hear that the organization's leadership is committed to it.

The best way to commit senior leadership to the process is by having them attend some of the meetings. Having the CEO of the organization come to a department variation-reduction meeting, for example, says a lot to the physicians at the meeting. It also shows the leadership exactly what the process is all about. Watching how the data is presented in its nonjudgmental one-down approach, and seeing how physicians respond to the data and the approach, is extremely important to cultural change.

In most medical organizations, just below senior leadership are a number of physician leaders who are responsible for the day-to-day functioning of the organization. Whether they are called medical directors or department chiefs, these are key people in getting a variation-reduction project to work. They typically are also the busiest people in an organization, and adding one more thing to their plates is sometimes very difficult. What we ask of these operational leaders is not to actually do the process of variation reduction, but rather to just be aware of it and actively support it.

These physician leaders are your go-to people when you run into roadblocks. For example, when a particular specialty that you're working with is giving you a hard time scheduling a meeting, you can go to these operational leaders and ask them to exert pressure to get the meeting set. Most of the time we did not need to exert pressure on the specialists, but it's good to have these people in your corner when you need them.

PHYSICIAN ENGAGEMENT

Physicians must be at the center of any variation-reduction project. As I've already mentioned, for all the talk about patient-driven care, the physician is still the one to order the test, prescribe the medication, and perform the procedure. Only physicians can develop the standards of care that are appropriate for our own communities. At PAMF, we found that the best way to engage physicians in general was to recruit physician thought leaders as what we call "enthusiastic champions."

The use of the word "champion" in the variation-reduction project was deliberate. A champion is a person who defends, supports, and promotes something. A champion is someone who has a degree of excellence and achievement in a given area. The variation-reduction team wanted to recruit people who thought of themselves in this manner and supported the idea of variation. Building the word "enthusiastic" into the term was deliberate, too. The champions we recruit have high energy levels and enjoy the variation-reduction process. They like the challenge of the meetings, and they celebrate with their colleagues when a standard is set. Enthusiasm is contagious and an upbeat variation-reduction team increases the likelihood of a successful variation-reduction project.

Initially, we were undecided about whether the variation-reduction champions actually needed to be physicians. We thought that perhaps we could use some of the staff in the quality improvement office, because they had a lot of experience in interacting with physicians, dealing with data, and creating guidelines. So we experimented: we set up some teams led by physicians and some led by the non-physician quality-improvement staff. Within a short period of time, it became painfully obvious that the staff-led teams weren't getting anywhere; the physician-led teams, on the other hand, moved ahead rapidly, creating and spreading the standards.

Why did the use of non-physicians as variation-reduction leaders not work? What we were asking physicians to do was not dissimilar from what insurance companies and other regulatory agencies have been asking for many years. This type of outside pressure had always been resisted by physicians as unwarranted interference with the physician-patient relationship. Our variation-reduction team was asking physicians to look at the way they practice medicine, especially in areas where there was no evidence-based medicine but rather only expert opinion. Having that request come from administration and staff rubbed physicians the wrong way—a familiar wrong way.

When the variation-reduction process is led by a physician champion, a different dynamic is set up. No longer is an outside agency pressuring physicians; no longer is the predominant feeling one of judgment. Rather, your colleague, who works down the hall, is asking, "Why do you do it that way?" The variation-reduction physician champion promulgates the idea that all of our specialists want to do the right thing for our patients. The goal is to find what just what that right thing is.

After that, physicians' natural competitive urges kick in and work to your favor: all physicians had to be in the top part of their classes in college to get into medical school. They had to be in the top part of their medical-school classes to get the good internships. And so on. When physicians see that a particular behavior is ranking them "low" on whatever scale they're looking at, they'll come to you asking, "What can I do about this?" All physicians believe that they are "above-average." (In this respect they apparently identify with Garrison Keillor's Lake Wobegon.) When you show them data that indicate they're not, they are powerfully driven to regain their status.

At PAMF, we mainly focus our variation-reduction efforts on specialists. So our next questions were: Should variation-reduction champions be specialists themselves? Or can Primary Care physicians be variation-reduction champions? We found that it was more a question of who was available, respected, and enthusiastic, rather than the type of physicians they were. Both specialists and Primary Care physicians can act as variation-reduction champions, and both work equally well. After all, because specialists are knowledgeable, typically, in only one area, they are at no advantage over the Primary Care physicians in their knowledge of other specialties. And, indeed, we have had a few instances where the variation-reduction champion was a specialist, and was leading that department's specialty in the variation-reduction project. It did not seem to make the process go any more smoothly than when the variation-reduction champion was a Primary Care physician. The more important attribute of variation-reduction champions is that they be considered good clinicians by their peers. Physicians who are recognized by their peers as the doctors they'd want to see are the physicians you want to have as variation-reduction champions.

Most PAMF physicians are based at one of three major locations. At each of these three sites, we have both Primary Care and specialty physicians; so, as we went to ramp up the variation-reduction project from a pilot (which was based at just one of the sites), we knew it was important to get physician champions at all three of our sites and that they be very familiar with the local physicians and their personalities.

The initial three variation-reduction champions were identified and appointed by the organization's leadership. Subsequent variation-reduction team members have been recruited through an open process. When there are openings for new variation-reduction champions, we send out a notice through E-mail, voice mail, and other types of communication such as a newsletter and a physician blog. All applicants are given a detailed job description plus information about the variation-reduction process. We ask as many of the variation-reduction team members as possible to speak to the applicants by phone or in person, and then the whole team meets to rank the applicants. In the most recent round of recruitment, we had two slots and 15 applicants. We decided to have a group interview of five of the applicants and came away with two highly qualified variation-reduction champions.

Over time, we've come to realize the common characteristics of successful variation-reduction champions: they already have some experience with process improvement, they have worked with physicians in a team setting, and they are considered good clinicians. What they often do not have is knowledge of database management, advanced skills in the use of spreadsheets, or experience in graphing data for presentation. No matter: these skills, while important to a variation-reduction champion, are something that we can teach.

Robust data, a workable group structure, organizational commitment, and physician engagement: do you need all four? I would argue that you do; how much of each depends on your local conditions. Robust data are necessary but not sufficient for the variation-reduction process to flourish. Your group structure must allow for the sharing of information; organizational commitment and physician engagement are essential for change that's deep and abiding.

◆ ◆ ◆

This first chapter of Part III introduced the minimum conditions you'll need to foster variation reduction. The remaining chapters walk you through the practical decisions you'll need to make to create and implement a variation-reduction project. Chapter 12 provides tips for gathering and analyzing your data; Chapter 13 shows you how to use that data to measure and communicate variation. Chapter 14 discusses the practicalities of implementing variation-reduction: holding meetings with physicians and creating and implementing a standard of care. Chapter 15 describes some of the common problems you may encounter in dealing with difficult specialties.

CHAPTER 12

Working with Data

This chapter is about how to work with data—not just what we did with our data, but what you'll need to do with yours. You'll need to gather information from a targeted group of physicians who generate lots of patient data. You'll need to make sure that the data you gather is comparable and that you attribute it consistently.

Not surprisingly, you're likely to experience variation in the way you'll need to work with your data. This variation is expected—and warranted—because not all the groups of physicians who will want to participate in variation reduction will have the same resources.

START WITH TARGETED GROUPS OF PHYSICIANS

When you begin a variation-reduction project, start with one or a few targeted groups of physicians—groups small enough to be easy to interact with, but large enough to generate measurable variation.

At PAMF, we chose to concentrate on the variation of our specialists rather than Primary Care. Willie Sutton, the famous bank robber, is reported to have said that he robbed banks "because that's where the money is." Likewise, we looked at the specialists because that's where the cost is: specialists, for the most part, make the determinations about which procedures patients will undergo, which surgeries they will have, and, more often than not, under what circumstances they will be hospitalized.

Other factors make dealing with specialists a better idea than dealing with Primary Care physicians when starting a variation-reduction project. The first is the obvious: most groups have far fewer specialists than Primary Care physicians. PAMF has about 1000 physicians in our organization, half of whom are Primary Care providers. Even our largest specialty group, the OB/GYN Department, has only 75 providers, and most of our specialty departments are much smaller. Some are as small as 5 or 6 physicians; more often, there are about a dozen physicians in each specialty.

Having to deal with only about a dozen physicians at a time makes scheduling meetings much easier than trying to deal with hundreds or even dozens of Primary Care physicians, even if you're dealing with only one site. It also allows you to have all the physicians of most specialties in the room at the same time, which is key, because it's optimal for everyone in a department to be exposed to the variation-reduction data together.

A second benefit in using specialist data is that specialists deal with fewer issues on a given day than is typical for Primary Care providers. In fact, it was quite revealing to both the variation-reduction team and the specialists themselves to see how often they were all seeing patients with the same problem. In a typical month, all the Urologists saw dozens of patients with kidney stones, all the Allergists saw dozens of patients with allergic rhinitis, all the Pulmonologists saw dozens of patients with chronic-obstructive pulmonary disease, and so on. The fact that each specialist saw large numbers of similar patients made it easier for us to start the discussion about the variation.

A third factor making our specialists good subjects for a variation-reduction project is that not only are the specialists seeing the same type of patients (at least based on their diagnoses), they are also being fed by the same group of Primary Care physicians. For the most part, the way our Primary Care physicians refer a patient to a specialist is by referring the patient to the department, not to the specific specialist. Using this referral procedure, urgent referrals go to the on-call specialist and patients with non-urgent conditions get the earliest available regular appointment. Both of these referral patterns create similar patient panels for each of our specialists. At PAMF, it's fairly rare for physicians to have such specialized practices that the Primary Care providers refer them to directly. Even those physicians with particular procedural skills are not, for the most part, directly referred to; rather, their specialist colleagues refer patients to them if they think that the particular procedural skill is required in treating those particular patients.

A good example of this referral procedure is in the Dermatology Department, where we have 30 Dermatologists, only two of who are trained in performing Moh's surgery for skin cancers. When Primary Care refers the patient to Dermatology for a suspected skin cancer, the patient is seen by the next-available Dermatologist, and if the Dermatologist makes the diagnosis of skin cancer and determines that the patient is a candidate for Moh's surgery, the Dermatologist refers the patient to one of the two specialists within the department who do that procedure.

A fourth reason it's easier to gather data on specialists than on Primary Care physicians is that specialists generally perform procedures; encounters with Primary Care physicians are mainly office visits. Now, I realize that Primary Care physicians do a lot more than just see patients in the office, but their variation is complicated and some of their data, such as pharmacy utilization, is inconsistently available.

When we discuss variation in primary care, the issues are often ambiguous. When dealing with a common problem such as hypertension, for example, factors in variation include how often the physicians see the patients, how many tests they order, how often they refer to specialists, what kinds of medication they prescribe, and what level of office visit is necessary to treat a specific complaint. The conversation frequently degenerates into a "how to code" discussion rather than a discussion of variation in how patients are treated. It's just harder to make the case to Primary Care physicians that they should concentrate on their variation in clinical decision making.

Does this mean that if you are strictly a Primary Care group, you cannot do variation reduction? Of course not, but you will face some issues that are less problematic when dealing with specialists. You can adapt some of the lessons we learned about dealing with specialists.

First, don't look at all your Primary Care physicians (PCPs); begin with a subset. A reasonable number is between 10 and 15 PCPs. This relatively small number makes it easy logistically to schedule the meetings while including enough providers to see real variation.

Second, create some sample data sets. In Primary Care a larger amount of the variation may be warranted; you'll need to deal with that first, especially when deciding how to adjust for the difference in provider panels.

(See the next section of this chapter.) The data for providers with patients who are all young and healthy will look different than data for those with a Geriatrics practice. Adjusting by age and sex is a traditional methodology to account for these differences.[31]

What about groups that do have specialists but have only one or two physicians in each specialty? It's pretty hard to see variation in a Rheumatology Department of one. Still, you can look at two Rheumatologists and see if there's variation. We started our variation-reduction process by looking at a group of only five ENT physicians. Fortunately, virtually all specialties have national organizations that typically create guidelines for care to support their members. The American College of Cardiology (ACC) is particularly active in this area. It has created appropriate-use criteria for both cardiac imaging procedures as well as cardiac surgeries.[32] Even a single Cardiologist could be compared to the ACC's appropriate-use criteria.

GATHER A LOT OF PATIENT DATA

Why is working with small numbers of patients a problem when discussing variation reduction? It means that you have to spend time and effort to continuously adjust your data to compensate for individual risk factors.

In the managed care era of the 1990s, health plans and medical groups worked hard to risk-adjust patient populations, spurred by their desire to have a scientific method for paying Primary Care physicians to care for panels of patients. Research identified three ways to make panels of patients comparable. For large panels (100 or more patients), the sheer number of patients tends to even out variations in the population; just by statistical chance, each large panel can be expected to have patients with similar risks to other large panels. Moderately sized panels (20 to 99 patients) can be risk-adjusted based on just age and sex: because it's known that the very young and the very old cost the most to care for, and woman cost more to care for than men, panels with more woman and patients who are younger or older can be expected to require more costly care. For the smallest panels of patients (fewer than 20 patients), it's necessary to take into account not only age and sex, but co-morbid conditions: you can't expect that all patients have one and only one complaint, and a patient who comes in with multiple medical problems along with the primary complaint is more difficult to treat because the physician has to take into account all the other conditions.

What most of the insurance companies have tried to do in the past, and what Aetna was doing with its Symmetry process, was to say, "OK. We'll take into account all these extra variables and weight each case a little bit differently so we can make good predictions even with smaller numbers of cases." Basically, the Symmetry process was an attempt to get around the issue of the small numbers. But when the data set is very small, the weighting doesn't resolve the issue because of the impact of random factors. Sometimes a patient without any of the common risk factors experiences multiple complications, a problem that—while unexpected in the given case—is expected to occur in a percentage of cases. Because these events occur randomly, a small panel for a particular problem might contain that one random event that is very expensive. Until a given physician sees enough patients for statistical significance, that one random event makes the physician's average cost for treating the condition seem very high in comparison to supposedly similar panels.

The subset of Aetna's data regarding the treatment of congestive heart failure at PAMF, for example, held only five cases. One of the four Cardiologists had not even one case in the Aetna data set; the remaining three had two cases each, at most. All could point to a particular episode and say something like, "Well, I remember this particular patient. She was really very difficult. It was a very unusual case, and you can't hold that against me." And, quite frankly, the Cardiologists were correct on that.

For all these reasons, PAMF quickly abandoned the Aetna data set. Our own approach was to say, "Well, let's not worry about the small numbers. Let's get big numbers, because we know our physicians are taking care of large numbers of patients." When you have a large number of cases—and in some of our variation-reduction projects, we had well in excess of 100 to 200 cases for every physician—it just works out that everybody gets the one or two bad cases, and the expected variation loses its importance because everybody has a "bad" case once in a while and everybody gets a few patients who are at high risk.

I say that it "just works out" that panels become comparable, but we didn't accept the idea on faith; instead, we tested the hypothesis. Our data analysts told us that having specialty panels of 50 or more patients for the same condition produced better statistical results than adjusting the panels by age, sex, or co-morbidity. Still, we felt obligated to convince ourselves and our specialist colleagues that risk adjustment was not necessary. So we did risk-adjust a number of data sets.

When we were looking at the Allergists and their use of skin testing in the diagnosis of allergic rhinitis, we thought that chronic sinusitis or asthma might be co-morbid conditions that would change the way a physician treated patients. When we developed adjusted panel sizes and weighted averages for the cost of treating patients with the co-morbid conditions, however, we found that these adjustments did not change the fact of variation between physicians. We then adjusted the Allergists' panels based on age/sex and again found that the adjustment did not explain the variation.

Despite this confirmation, other groups, such as the Internal Medicine physicians, had us age/sex–adjust their very large panels (ranging from 500 to 2000 patients) when we were looking at variation in the way they treated hypertension. Again, the overall pattern of variation remained the same.[33]

Although age/sex adjustment did not remove the Internists' variation, they were sure that some other confounding factor must exist, so they asked the variation-reduction team to take into account co-morbid conditions associated with hypertension: diabetes and hyperlipidemia (elevated cholesterol). So we reran the data. We called the patients with hypertension, diabetes, and hyperlipidemia the "triad" patients and those with hypertension alone the "non-triad" patients. When we separated the triad patients from the non-triad patients, the variation pattern was exactly the same: physicians who had a higher cost per patient with their triad patients also had a higher cost per patient with their non-triad patients. Convinced by our willingness to perform traditional risk adjustment for their data, the Internists were willing to move forward and look at their own decision making as the source of the variation.

Through our experiments, we found that when we were dealing with more than 30 to 50 patients in a physician panel for a specific diagnosis, each physician generally had one or two patients with significant co-morbid conditions. Each specialist had a few patients at high risk, with multiple co-morbid conditions, but most patients were of average risk, without co-morbid conditions. While including these patients at high risk did increase the cost of caring for the group as a whole, the increase occurred in all specialists' panels. Whether we eliminated these patients from the data set or kept them in the mix, the variation was still there.

How did we go about getting large numbers of cases for each physician? The simplest answer is that we decided to use all of our patients. Rather than a portion of our patients, say the patients from just one health plan, or just the patients with HMO insurance, or just the patients insured by Medicare, we would look at all the encounters for all of our patients. It turned out that our business office had a data warehouse of all of our encounter submissions. It was routinely collecting this information so that it could bill the various health plans and Medicare for our services and track whether we were getting paid properly for our services. This apparently is a very common business practice for most medical groups. In fact, even solo practitioners do exactly the same thing; they need some way of tracking whether they've been paid by an insurance company. That meant that we didn't have to do any special collection to develop our variation-reduction data; it was obtained solely from the encounter data.

So, we had a data warehouse where all this information was stored, and our IT staff created a front end to the data warehouse so I could easily query it without having to do any programming. (This front end also allows me to pull information out without risking damage to the original data.) It became a very simple process to say, "OK. We're going to look at all the Cardiologists and the patients they saw for congestive heart failure." We knew who the Cardiologists were, and we knew that the diagnosis code for congestive heart failure was 429.00, so we could query the database for all encounters by a given Cardiologist where the diagnosis code was 429.00. As we grew familiar with the front-end query system, our ability to create complex queries grew.

Using this system, numerical data for each specialist jumped rather dramatically from when we were dealing only with the Aetna data. For example, now, when we used data from all our patients, we had data on well over 100 cases of congestive heart failure per Cardiologist. When I went back to the Cardiologists with the new data, and they saw the number of cases that were being analyzed, it became easier for them to accept that, yes, they did have a bad case with Mrs. Jones, but they also had quite a number of standard cases, and that everybody had a "Mrs. Jones" in their group of patients.

When you are starting a variation-reduction project, you'll need some sample data sets to show physicians how the process works. Pick sample topics such that you'll have large numbers of patients for each physician. This means choosing common clinical problems. For general surgery, this might mean inguinal hernia repairs or removal of gallbladders; for Gastroenterology, it will likely mean colonoscopies or upper endoscopies. These sample data sets are just examples of what type of data you can supply to your physicians. Letting the physicians themselves choose the topic for examination is key to engaging them in the variation-reduction process.

What if you have data available only from patients with HMO insurance? This limitation does not mean you cannot start a variation-reduction program, but it does mean that you'll have the problems of small numbers of patients for each physician. One way to increase the numbers is to review a longer time frame than the year we typically use. If you have data over a five-year period, use it. (You may need to convert the charges to a standard charge master because it would have been very common in recent years to see charges change each year for the same service.)

FILTER DOWN TO DATA THAT'S COMPARABLE

In the pilot phase of our variation-reduction project, we looked at all patients seen for a particular diagnosis, making no distinction between old and new patients. But we found that this choice distorted the conclusions we reached from our data. For example, ENT physicians seeing new patients for chronic sinusitis might appropriately do fiber-optic nasal endoscopy, a procedure that we know drives up the cost of treating such patients. Because new ENT physicians have more open spaces on their schedules than established ENT physicians, they see relatively more of the new patients and can be expected to do more nasal endoscopies during the data-gathering period than physicians who were following patients over a period of years and had done the procedure years before. Treating all of these encounters the same would lead to the incorrect conclusion that new ENTs' treatment for chronic sinusitis shows unwarranted variation.

Because this issue pertains for lots of different disease entities, you must, in essence, front-load the data-gathering process. When patients first come in, they have a lot of testing done, because you're establishing a baseline for them; then, as you follow them along, you may request additional tests, but you don't have to go through that whole initial evaluation again.

So, as we moved from the pilot phase to system-wide implementation of variation reduction, we wanted to think about a way of separating the new-patient problem from the old-patient problem. And one of the things that we realized was that, in general, PAMF specialists were seeing a lot of new patients—not necessarily patients who were new to our system, but patients with a new clinical entity that needed evaluation by one of our specialists. If we filtered the data to look only at the evaluation and treatment of these new patients, we still had large numbers of patients for each of our doctors. By concentrating on the new patients, we eliminated the spurious variation caused by the difference between the open practices and the mature practices.

Doing so was important, because to get anywhere with variation reduction, you must supply physicians with believable data. It is truly amazing how often physicians will focus with laser-like precision on a single flaw in the data and then condemn the entire data set as utterly useless. One of the ways to avoid this fate is to set up the data criteria to be as fair, consistent, and comparable as possible. Using only new patients is a good example. While we acknowledge that each patient can be different, patients sent to a specialist for a particular diagnosis will have certain commonalities. You can use this fact to level the playing field initially and then see over time how each specialist handles the clinical problem.

Looking at only new patients also allowed us to standardize another variable: the length of time the patient was seen by the specialist. We decided to look at data delivered by PAMF within a five-year period of care. For any given patient, we examined one year of data beginning with the day that the specialist was first consulted about the patient. So, for example, over a five-year period, we looked for the all the initial encounters in which an Oncologist saw a patient for breast cancer by looking for the Current Procedural Terminology (CPT) code for a new-patient visit or new consultation. When we queried this filtered database, we found more than 800 new patients with breast cancer. During this time, PAMF had 10 Oncologists, all of whom had seen at least 50 new patients with breast cancer, and some of whom had seen more than 100. Having large panels for all the Oncologists made the variation data realistic when we presented it.

For purposes of comparability, we chose to measure variation as cost per patient per diagnosis per specialist. Our decision to measure by charges for procedures was a matter of convenience. We were well aware that our charges had nothing to do with either our true revenues or what the patient would be responsible for paying. However, because the organization, not the individual physician, sets the charges, we knew that as long as we kept the charge master fixed for any procedure, we could easily show variation among the physicians. We also hoped that if the standards worked, we could easily show the effect of each standard by decreased average charges per patient. We could just as easily have used work relative value units (RVUs) as our measure, but it seemed easier to deal in dollars rather than the abstraction of RVUs. We had no serious complaints from our specialists about using the average cost per patient as a measure of variation.

The use of charges did present one problem: every year we changed our charge master, so from one year to the next, the charge for the same proce-dure might be different. We needed to adjust the charge master so that we could compare the average charge per patient from one year to the next. That entailed a certain degree of complexity, especially when dealing with surgical modifiers, but with the help of some skilled database managers we overcame the problem.

The other variable that we needed to adjust was length of treatment. We had arbitrarily chosen one year from the time of the consultation, but some specialties asked that we vary the length of time. The Neurosurgeons, for example, indicated that it was not uncommon for them to treat a patient with back pain conservatively for at least a year before deciding to operate, so they asked us to give them two-year data. On the other hand, the Oncolo-gists felt that six months of data was enough to give them a good idea if their standard was appropriate. Our methodology was flexible enough to accommodate a range of requests.

Another piece of the comparability puzzle was classifying a patient's treatment by its relation to the date when the standard was put in place.

We looked to see whether the patient was seen for the new-patient/new-consultation visit before or after the standard was set. Even if most of the one-year data were in the post-standard time frame, if the consult was done before the standard was announced, we counted that patient as a pre-standard patient. We were then able to compare the average cost per patient pre-standard to the average cost per patient post-standard. The difference between those two multiplied by the number of patients seen in the post-standard period is the savings to the patient attributed to the new standard. For example, if the average cost per patient in the pre-standard period was $1000, and the average cost per patient post-standard was $500, and 10 patients were seen during that post-standard period, the total savings would be $500 times 10, or $5000. (We did make the assumption that if the patient had been seen before the institution of the standard, the patient would have had the same average cost as the pre-standard period.)

ATTRIBUTE THE DATA CONSISTENTLY

To measure variation by physician, you'll need to be able to attribute the cost to treat a patient to the responsible physician—typically a problem in any system that looks at individual physician variation. Again, the exclusive use of the new patient encounter helps with this problem. Our variation-reduction team decided, and our physicians agreed, that the first specialist who saw the patient for that problem was the patient's primary specialist and we attributed all the cost for the care of the patient for that particular problem to that initial consultant.

(We did find that a small number of patients were seen first by one specialist and then by a second; we kept the attribution to the first specialist anyway. When we presented this methodology, our specialists were comfortable with our attribution schema. They recognized that instances of patients seeking more than one specialty consultation were rare, and that this was probably the best way of attributing the patient to the individual specialist.)

In the case of our Oncology Department, for example, we attributed a new patient to the Oncologist who first saw the patient, and we set the initiating date as the date of the new-patient visit/new-patient consultation. We then looked at all encounters within the specialty for the diagnosis of breast cancer, tagging those that were 365 days or less after the date of the initial consultation. In addition, we developed encounter tables that included ancillary services such as imaging and laboratory linked to that same diagnosis. Because the patient's primary Oncologist was responsible for the care of the patient for breast cancer, and the Oncologist should be in contact with Primary Care colleagues to ensure that appropriate studies were being done, we and the specialists decided that even if a test was ordered by Primary Care, it should still be attributed to the Oncologist. It didn't matter who ordered the test, only that the test was ordered after the initial consultation and was appropriate for the diagnosis.

Using this methodology, we were able to attribute total PAMF charges to each Oncologist and to divide that number by the total number of new patients, giving us the average cost per patient for breast cancer attributed to that Oncologist. (We eliminated from study any Oncologist who had only a few cases, typically a vacation fill-in or some other type of part-time physician.)

This decision to attribute the patient to the first specialist allowed us to avoid many instances of inconsistent attribution and spurious variation. In the question of referrals for Moh's surgery, for example, had we had looked at occurrences of the procedure in isolation, we would have found only the two physicians who performed the surgery; none of the other Dermatologists would have appeared in the data. Instead, our variation-reduction methodology attributes the patient to the Dermatologist who recommends the surgery, not the specialist who performs it. That way, should we find any variation in referrals for the surgery, that variation is real. Our initial variation data for Dermatology showed exactly that: that some Dermatologists refer for Moh's surgery more frequently than others. This information became the impetus for the Dermatologists to create their own standard of care on the treatment of basal-cell carcinomas.

Despite the many advantages of filtering the data by attributing the physician by new-patient visit, there are times when this technique does not fit the clinical condition. For example, how could we handle singular events such as encounters in Urgent Care or chronic conditions such as diabetes? We developed two additional strategies for filtering attribution data: a procedure-based methodology that tracks what was done and a frequency-based methodology that tracks who saw the patient for a given condition most often. The procedure-based strategy works best when the procedure is a unique event: a gallbladder can be removed only once. In such a case, the primary surgeon becomes the attributed physician, the date of surgery is the date of record, and services before and after that date can easily be tallied.

The frequency-based method is often required for Primary Care, where it's fairly common for patients to switch PCPs and come to the first visit with a list of problems that have already been diagnosed by other physicians—which means that the first visit is not for diagnosis, but for continuation of ongoing therapy. In this case, the PCP who sees the patient most often becomes the attributed physician. While face-to-face encounters currently take place as office visits, future encounters may be virtual visits—an additional challenge for any attribution strategy.

◆ ◆ ◆

Working with data is necessary to the variation-reduction process. The better you understand how the data are gathered, the more confident you can be when facing physicians who doubt its validity. Make sure you understand the target group of physicians, the volume of patient data gathered, how the data were made comparable, and how the data were attributed to each physician. Then you can concentrate on analyzing and communicating the variation.

CHAPTER 13

Analyzing and Communicating Variation

Now that you've gathered a robust amount of accurate, comparable, and attributable data, how do you analyze the data to discover variation? How do you use the data to provide your physicians with an understandable picture of how they are practicing? And how do you do it without offending them?

None of these problems is trivial: Because physicians are scientists as well as clinicians, you must use scientifically defensible methods to analyze the data. Because physicians must really believe that unwarranted variation exists before they'll create the standards to reduce it, you must present the results of your analysis in a way that's compelling. And because physicians must be willing to engage with the data in order to believe it, you can't risk offending them in the process.

ANALYZING VARIATION

To carry out variation reduction, you need data analysis that provides an accurate reflection of how your physicians are practicing. For this kind of analysis, you need data that will stand up to scrutiny, but you don't need data that meet the kind of statistical reliability necessary for publishing a paper in the medical literature. The purpose of the analysis is to start the discussion; data and their analysis are a necessary but not sufficient component of the variation-reduction process.

Almost immediately after we started this work, we found there was a certain amount of excitement, even anxiety, among the physicians in the room regarding our results. Would we be publishing them? Some physicians wanted to know because they felt that publishing this information would add to the general knowledge. Others with a more jaundiced eye wanted to know if publication was our main reason for doing the project. I told both sets of physicians that our interest was in improving the care to our patients and making PAMF more affordable for them. Publishing our results was secondary, and we would not even consider it for a number of years. (Indeed, although we've presented our results at a number of conferences, we've yet to submit them for publication in any medical journal.) I think it was important for us to make that statement to our physicians: that we were there to help them provide more value to the patient, not to use them as experimental fodder for our own personal or professional gain. I believe this stance helped us establish a degree of credibility and acceptability with our physicians. Had we gone about the projects in a more traditional, scientific way, we might have been able to publish a number of papers, but we would not have gained the engagement of our physicians as quickly.

Getting people to accept the fact that we were not looking for—and would not provide—scientifically provable, statistically significant changes was difficult. As we spread the variation-reduction methodology to all of Sutter Health, the strategy to measure change became a significant issue. But the goal for variation reduction is to increase for patients the value of the care they are receiving. We want to maintain or increase the quality and decrease the cost. Can such a clinical process realistically be held to the standards of a strict scientific method? Since you really are not performing a formal experiment with control groups in a controlled situation, I think the issue of statistical significance is a distraction. What we really need to measure are two things: Have we maintained or improved our quality of care? Have we decreased its cost?

To get to work on measuring variation, you need as complete a list of the relevant clinical encounters as possible. Each encounter must include the name of the patient, the procedure done, the performing physician, and the date of service. While you may not be able to gather all the relevant encounters, it's important to be consistent in the data you use. For example, some of our outpatient surgeries take place at hospitals where the Anesthesiologists are not PAMF physicians, so we have no billing records for those services; if the same procedure is done at a PAMF surgery center, the Anesthesiologist is a PAMF physician who will generate an encounter for that service. Because we know that we have inconsistent records of anesthesia encounters, we eliminate all anesthesia encounters from our analyses.

Another issue you'll need to deal with is making sure you create a standard charge master. If you are looking at several years of data, your fees may have changed from year to year. You'll need to standardize those fees so that variations noted are not simply because of changes in charge masters.

Spreadsheets and summary or "pivot" tables are great tools to organize and work with these types of data. Microsoft's Excel spreadsheet program is probably the most commonly used program of this type; if you're unfamiliar with it, a quick Internet search will yield all the tutorials you'll need to learn how to use spreadsheets to generate the pivot tables that not only summarize the charges but can organize your data in ways that can help you understanding the causes of the variation.

The first metric you'll need to create for the specialty under discussion is the average charge per patient for each specialist. For example, if the topic under discussion is treatment of kidney stones by Urologists, you'll add up all the Urology charges attributed to each Urologist and divide that total by the number of new patients seen for kidney stones by the attributed Urologist.

Start by creating a spreadsheet containing all Urology encounters for kidney stones. (See Table 1.)

Then use a pivot table to draw from the master table only those patients who are in your kidney-stone registry—that is, who had a new-patient or new-consultation visit with one of the Urologists. Table 2 shows a pivot table for Urologist-attributed encounters for kidney stones.

Attribute each kidney-stone encounter to the Urologist who did the initial consult. (At PAMF, we look for all kidney-stone encounters done on the day of the initial encounter and within the next 365 days.) Total the charges attributed to each Urologist, then find the average charge for each Urologist by dividing the total charges by number of attributed patients:

	A	B	C	D	E	F	G	H	I
		Performing				Procedure	Procedure		
1	Division	Provider Code	Procedure Co	Procedure Name	Modific	Date	Charge Amt	Units	MRN
4	PALO ALTO DIVISION	765	55840	PROSTATECTOMY RETROPUBIC RAD W/WO NERVE-SPAR		2007-01-03	5768	1	7523640
17	SANTA CRUZ DIVISION	6639	99243	OUTPT CONSULTATION,L3	57	2007-01-12	339	1	4472197
18	SANTA CRUZ DIVISION	6639	81000	URINALYSIS, NONAUTOMATED, WITH MICROSCOPY		2007-01-12	24.4	1	4472197
19	PALO ALTO DIVISION	765	9999	POST-OP VISIT		2007-01-15	0	1	7523640
20	PALO ALTO DIVISION	765	A4344	CATH INDWELLING 2-WAY SILICONE [FOLEY]		2007-01-25	31	1	4597738
21	PALO ALTO DIVISION	765	51798	US POST-VOID RESID URINE/BLAD CAP MEAS NON-IMAGI	AG	2007-01-25	150	1	4597738
37	PALO ALTO DIVISION	765	99244	CONSULT OUT-PT LEVEL 4	25	2007-01-25	554	1	4597738
41	PALO ALTO DIVISION	765	A4344	CATH INDWELLING 2-WAY SILICONE [FOLEY]		2007-01-29	31	1	5510359
55	PALO ALTO DIVISION	765	99211	OV MINIMAL SERVICE	25	2007-01-29	75	1	5510359
77	PALO ALTO DIVISION	765	51702	INSERT TEMP INDWELL BLADDER CATH SIMPLE [FOLEY]	AG	2007-01-29	402	1	5510359
78	PALO ALTO DIVISION	765	A4358	URINARY LEG OR ABDOMEN BAG		2007-01-29	10	1	5510359
79	SANTA CRUZ DIVISION	6639	99212	OFFICE/OUTPT VISIT,EST,L2	25	2007-01-31	107	1	4472197
80	SANTA CRUZ DIVISION	6639	81000	URINALYSIS, NONAUTOMATED, WITH MICROSCOPY		2007-01-31	24.4	1	4472197
81	SANTA CRUZ DIVISION	6639	52000	CYSTOSCOPY.		2007-01-31	576.05	1	4472197
232	PALO ALTO DIVISION	765	52000	CYSTOSCOPY (SEP PROC)	AG	2007-02-09	825	1	4597738
233	PALO ALTO DIVISION	765	99213	OV EST PT LEVEL 3	25	2007-02-09	155	1	4597738
234	PALO ALTO DIVISION	765	9999	POST-OP VISIT		2007-02-12	0	1	7523640
235	CAMINO DIVISION	1447	99212	OV EST PT LEVEL 2		2007-02-21	104	1	483370
236	PALO ALTO DIVISION	765	9999	POST-OP VISIT		2007-02-22	0	1	7523640
237	CAMINO DIVISION	1447	99212	OV EST PT LEVEL 2		2007-02-22	104	1	1796581
238	PALO ALTO DIVISION	765	99213	OV EST PT LEVEL 3		2007-03-22	155	1	7052392
239	SANTA CRUZ DIVISION	6639	99243	OUTPT CONSULTATION,L3		2007-04-05	362.75	1	5505910
240	CAMINO DIVISION	1447	99212	OV EST PT LEVEL 2		2007-04-11	104	1	6244628
241	PALO ALTO DIVISION	765	99213	OV EST PT LEVEL 3		2007-04-16	155	1	7523640

TABLE 1. Excel Spreadsheet for Kidney-Stone Encounters

TABLE 2. Pivot Table Showing Total Urology New Patients at a Particular Urology Clinic

$$\text{Average Charge} = \frac{\text{Total Charges in Dollars}}{\text{Total Number of New Patients}}$$

	A	B	C	D
1	After Initiating Event	Yes		
2	Within 1 Year of Initiating Event	Yes		
3		Pre Standard	Post Standard	
4	Urologist	Sum of Charge Amt	Sum of Charge Amt	
5	3006	$1,793,922.95	$1,026,425.10	
6	3053	$2,897,304.90	$2,377,280.80	
7	3605	$423,133.88	$490,844.95	
8	5989	$845,538.10	$905,296.53	
9	40094	$429,165.38	$525,529.18	
10	40158	$747,037.83	$1,140,068.45	
11	11000104	$369,123.43	$304,532.30	
12	11000116	$601,049.60	$1,326,296.90	
13	11000205	$408,122.59	$425,590.10	
14	11000627	$533,581.76	$681,884.98	
15	Total	$9,047,980.42	$9,203,749.29	
16				

TABLE 3. Pre- and Post-Standard Pivot Table

The second metric you'll need to create has to do with patient charges before and after the "standard date"—that is, the date on which physicians put in place the new standard of care. At PAMF, we typically wait 6 to 12 months after implementation of a new standard before we try to see its effect. At that time we do another data pull. This time we attribute the patient not only to a specific specialist but also to whether the new-patient or new-consultation encounter took place before or after the standard date. Using the same process, we calculate the average charge for each specialist before and after the standard was implemented so that the specialists can see how the standard has affected their practice. Table 3 shows a pivot table that filters encounters to within one year of the initial event and aggregates into pre- and post-standard timeframes.

To determine the savings created by the standard, we calculate the difference between the average charge (AC) for all specialists in the pre-standard period and the average charge for all specialists in the post-standard period, then multiply the result by the number of new patients seen in the post-standard time frame:

Savings = (Pre-AC—Post-AC) × New Patients

(We assume that if the standard had not been put in place, the specialists would have treated new patients just as they were already treating existing patients.)

The third metric has to do with understanding what's causing the variation. To analyze this issue, we create pivot tables of the procedures, their

Count of Procedure Code		Total
09977	PRE OP VISIT	3
09999	POST-OP VISIT	43
50080	KIDNEY STONE REMOVAL UP TO 2CM	3
50081	KIDNEY STONE REMOVAL OVER 2CM	1
50394	INJ PYELOGRAPHY THRU NEPHRO/PYELO TUBE OR CATH	2
50395	INTRO RENAL PELVIS GUIDE W/DILATION PERCUT	4
50590	FRAGMENTING OF KIDNEY STONE	1
	LITHOTRIPSY EXTRACORPOREAL SHOCK WAVE	156
51701	INSERT NON-DWELL BLADDER CATH [FOR RESID URINE]	2
51702	INSERT TEMP INDWELL BLADDER CATH SIMPLE [FOLEY]	43
51798	MEASUREMENT PVR URIN&/BLADO CAP US NON-IMAG	1
	US POST-VOID RESID URINE/BLAD CAP MEAS NON-IMAGE	6
52000	CYSTOSCOPY [SEP PROC]	24
52005	CYSTOSCOPY W/URETERAL CATH	43
52204	CYSTOURETHROSCOPY W/BX(S)	1
52224	CYSTOSCOPY W/FULG OR MIN LESION TRMNT W/WO BX	1
52281	CYSTOSCOPY W CALIB/DILATE URETHRAL STRICT/STEN	1
52310	CYSTOSCOPY W FB/CALC/STENT RMVL SIMPLE	56
52318	LITHOLAPAXY CRUSH/FRAG CALC IN BLADDER COMPLEX	2
52330	CYSTOSCOPY W/MANIP W/O URETER CALC RMVL	15
52332	CYSTOSCOPY W/INDWELL URETERAL STENT INSERT	247
52344	CYSTOSCOPY W/URETEROSCOPY W/TX URET STRICT	1
52351	CYSTOSCOPY W/URETEROSCOPY DIAG	17
52352	CYSTOSCOPY W/CALC RMVL/MANIP [INCL URETER CATH]	16
52353	CYSTOSCOPY W/LITHOTRIPSY [INCL URETER CATH]	160
52601	TRANSURETHRAL ELECTRO SURG PROSTATE COMPLETE	1
53600	DILATE URETHRA STRICT BY SOUND/DILATOR MALE INIT	1
7442028	XRAY UROGRAPHY RETROGRADE W/WO KUB PROF COMP BO	5
74485	XRAY DILATION NEPHROSTOMY S & I [50395,53600.53621]	2
7600080	FLUOROSCOPY UP TO 1 HR MD TIME [SEP PROC] BO	2
76705	US ABDOMEN LIMITED	1
76775	US RETROPERITONEAL LIMITED	1
8100001	URINALYSIS, NONAUTOMATED, WITH MICROSCOPY	1
81001	AUTOMATED URINALYSIS W/ MICROSCOPY	3
	URINALYSIS AUTO W/MICROSCOPY [BACK OFFICE]	86
81002	URINALYSIS NON-AUTO W/O MICRO [BACK OFFICE]	28
81003	URINALYSIS AUTO W/O MICRO [BACK OFFICE]	202
90772	THER/PROPHYLACTIC/DIAG INJECTION SQ/IM-DEL 2009	1
93000	EKG ROUTINE COMPLETE	5
96372	TX/PROPHY/DX INJECTION SQ/IM	4
99024	POST OPERATIVE FOLLOW-UP VISIT	13
99201	OV NEW PT LEVEL 1	1
99202	OV NEW PT LEVEL 2	8
99203	OV NEW PT LEVEL 3	59
99204	OV NEW PT LEVEL 4	33

TABLE 4. Results from Pivot Table Sorted by CPT Codes

CPT codes, and the accumulated charges. (These are total charges, without regard to which specialists ordered the procedures.) What we're looking for is patterns. Fortunately, CPT codes are ordered in a logical manner: procedures that are similar are close to one another; office visits and hospital visits are grouped together. Table 4 shows a sample list of procedure codes from our Urology data set. (The full table has more than 80 rows.)

Depending on the clinical situation, we frequently add laboratory and/or imaging information into our analysis of variation. Lab and imaging are sometimes ordered by the treating specialists but often are ordered by PCPs. We look for all lab and imaging ordered on the registry patient whether ordered by the specialist or a PCP, and whether ordered before or after the specialty consult, but we count only tests ordered for the diagnosis under discussion. While including lab and imaging costs gives us a more complete picture of the variation, we know it's not the total cost of care because we don't have access to all the costs. In particular, we do not have access to the hospital costs.

Gathering these data has been useful; before we gathered data, we made mistakes. When we were looking at the Orthopedists' use of MRIs before knee arthroscopy, for example, we noted that two Orthopedists rarely ordered knee MRIs. But when we showed these data to a group of our Orthopedists, they did not believe the data; they said they knew that these two Orthopedists did, in fact, obtain knee MRIs before arthroscopy. When we went back to the data and expanded our search, we found that the missing MRIs had been ordered by the PCPs before the specialty consult. These two Orthopedists had told the PCPs to order the MRIs before the specialty consult so that the Orthopedists could discuss the MRIs with their patients at the time of the consult.

COMMUNICATING VARIATION

When we first began to show our data and analyses to our physicians, we showed them the pivot tables we'd created. For example, the pivot table in Table 5 shows data for 10 urologists, their average charge per patient, and the total number of new patients each physician saw in a given time period.

TABLE 5. Pivot Table Showing Urology Charges and Number of New Patients*

Urologist	Avg. charge per patient	No. of patients
A	$14,179	255
B	$10,678	422
C	$8865	61
D	$8039	114
E	$7784	156
F	$6727	155
G	$6318	109
H	$6213	99
I	$5592	49
J	$4940	142

* Note that the actual table would include the names of the individual physicians.

Although the data are accessible, they are not instantly understandable; nor are they compelling. They don't tell a story. So while we continued to make the tables available to physicians for their own analysis, we spent some time devising a way to present their

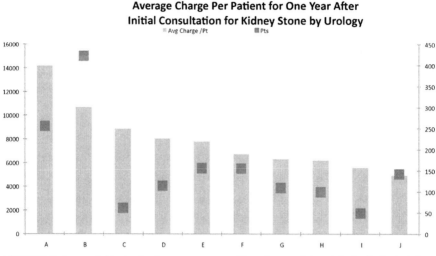

FIGURE 5. For each Urologist (here represented by a letter of the alphabet), the height of the bar represents the average cost of Urology charges per patient; the dot indicates the number of patients seen.

variation graphically. Eventually, we created a variation graph with two vertical axes. (See Figure 5.) The left vertical axis shows a scale for average charge, which is presented as a separate vertical bar for each physician. The right vertical axis shows a scale for the number of patients attributed to each physician, which is presented for each physician as a dot in line with that physician's bar.

With this kind of graphic presentation, the impact is immediate and profound. You easily can see what the variation-reduction team is talking about: a three- to four-fold variation is obvious in both average charge and number of patients per physician. Further, there's no relationship between each physician's average charge and the volume of patients the physician sees.

In some specialties, the variation we found was huge; in others, it was more modest. Over time, we learned how to make the variation more graphically apparent: don't use zero as the base of the vertical axis; instead, use a value just above the lowest value. For example, PAMF Pulmonologists have the least variation with regard to treatment of chronic asthma. When we began the two axes at zero (Figure 6), the variation in average charge was hard to see.

When we changed the scale by starting the left axis at $480 (Figure 7), in effect zooming in, the small variation became more apparent.

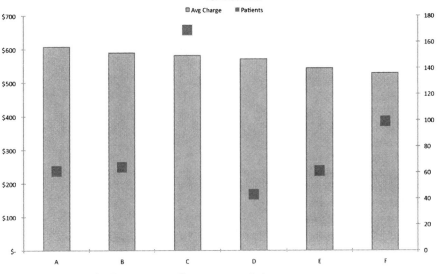

FIGURE 6. Vertical axis at zero; small apparent variation.

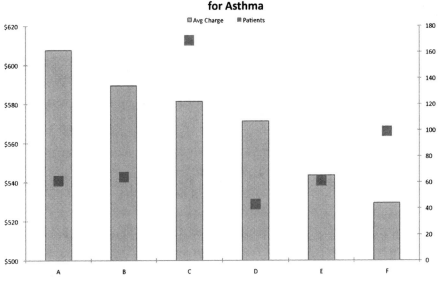

FIGURE 7. Vertical axis above zero; more visible variation.

When we want to show the variation on lab and imaging, we frequently use a stacked bar graph. (See Figure 8.) Stacked graphs are useful because they clearly show total charges as well as relative charges of each of the categories.

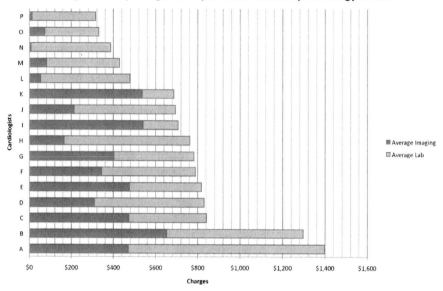

FIGURE 8. Stacked graph showing average charges attributed to each Cardiologist for imaging and lab procedures.

PAMF physicians are most interested in variation-reduction projects that are about value, not just cost. Recently, for example, the OB/GYN Department decided to examine its own compliance with the recommendation to screen for cervical cancer with Pap smears every three years. We looked at the interval between each Pap smear with the diagnosis of screening for cervical cancer (ICD-9 code V76xx).

With this project, determining attribution was trivial; it was the provider who performed the Pap smear. For each provider, we reported the percentage of Pap smears performed at the recommended screening interval, calculating the percentage by determining how many screening Pap smears were performed at the recommended interval divided by the total number of Pap smears performed for cervical cancer screening. The vertical bars in Figure 9 show that the OB/GYN providers vary in compliance: some providers comply in the 65% to 70% range while others are in compliance 80% to 95% of the time. The dots indicate the number of Pap smears done in total by each OB. From the path of the line, it appears the more pap smears a provider does the more likely that Pap smear will be out of compliance. At first this graph might seem strange. Typically the more

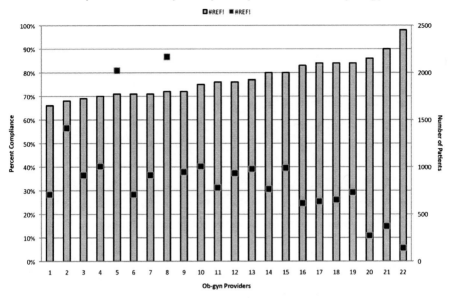

FIGURE 9. Each bar is the compliance rate for an OB/GYN provider. The dot graphs how many opportunities providers had to follow the standard. Most providers had more than 700 opportunities during this time frame to use or not use the standard.

procedures a physician does, the better the physician becomes at doing it. But that's not what's going on here. While the Pap smear may be perfect technically, the provider is performing it on a patient who does not need it. Those providers with high numbers of total Pap smears are apparently sticking to the old-school thinking that women need annual Pap smears, a concept outdated by the new three-year standard. These extra Pap smears are of little value to the patient not because they are of poor quality or high cost, but because they are unwarranted.

These graphs demonstrate the value of using the graphic display of data to combine information about cost with information about quality. By doing so, we can provide physicians with a better understanding of how their actions affect the value of their services to their patients.

PERSONALIZING VARIATION

Showing unblinded data is risky; at the beginning of our project, we worried that this information might embarrass some physicians to the point that they might not want to participate in the process. Anyone who has shown physicians data that compare one physician with another by name knows that you risk the kind of negative reaction that can stop any change effort in its tracks. So why risk putting the names of the physicians on the graphs in the first place?

We did consider partially blinding the data by assigning a code to each physician and giving the physicians only their own codes. That way, individual physicians would know where they stood on the graph, but they wouldn't know specifics about any of their colleagues' positions. We knew that other groups had done this type of semi-transparent data release for exactly this reason: they feared a backlash. This semi-transparent approach was also the way health plans release data to physicians, but presenting data in this manner usually does not get the desired behavior change.

I believe the main reason that the semi-transparent approach doesn't work is because it's too easy for physicians to revert to the claim that "my patients are sicker." Most physicians know what type of patients their colleagues care for. When we see differing results for a physician who has a similar panel of patients to ourselves, it's much harder to use the "my patients are sicker" justification.

Clear, attributed data foster physicians' discussion of their differences in clinical practice. So for our variation-reduction project, we decided that being totally transparent *within a specialty* was more important than the possibility of generating hurt feelings. We made it clear that we would not distribute variation graphs with physician names throughout the organization; only physicians' own departmental colleagues would see the unblinded data. We reasoned that this unblinded but limited release of data was low risk because some specialists already suspected (or knew) which of their colleagues showed the most variation.

(As the size of the departments grew, and especially as we started dealing with larger departments across wider geographic regions, the risk of offending increased, but by that time we had already established the value of the method, so physicians who joined the project entered already expecting this transparency.)

Most variation graphs had the same pattern. A few physicians had high cost per patient, a few had low cost per patient, and a larger number had about the same cost per patient. We especially wanted the high- and low-cost physicians to discuss their practice patterns that resulted in this variation. Without knowing who was where on the graph, how could we foster this discussion? Transparency was essential.

We also had a secret weapon, the one-down approach. By openly declaring that we did not understand the reasons for the variation, and without implying the presence of "good" or "bad" variation, our variation-reduction champions were able to defuse the negative reaction to the data. Further, we never even argued that the data were correct. Our standard one-down response to a challenge to the data was not to defend, but to ask how we could make it better. And we learned always to follow through with the data revisions that the physicians asked for.

Over the last three years, we've had only a few, if any, hostile reactions to our presentations of variation data, vindicating the one-down approach. It's hard to know which is more important: transparency or the one-down approach. We have no practical way of knowing. But it is our observation that the two techniques used together are greater than the sum of their parts.

In this chapter I have shown some of the ways we analyze variation at PAMF and communicate it to our PAMF physicians. I hope you can see from the examples that variation reduction does not require sophisticated data analysis. Rather, simple spreadsheet tools that are easily learned can produce the type of compelling data that will spur discussion. Remember, it not the data but the discussion among physicians of their different practices that leads to creation of a standard.

As you begin your variation-reduction program, it will probably seem that each new project brings a whole new set of challenges in how to analyze and present data. With time and some experience, however, patterns for data presentation appear. A variation-reduction project among one set of specialists on the use of one type of medication, for example, will most likely resemble the project you just completed with another set of specialists on another type of medication. As long as you provide data on variation to your physician colleagues, they can begin to understand and correct their unwarranted variation.

CHAPTER 14

Herding Cats

Now that you've gathered and analyzed the data, discovered variation in a department's work, and built compelling and personally identifiable visuals to show the physicians, it's time to hold a variation-reduction meeting—the first step in creating and implementing a local standard of care. I begin this chapter by discussing a couple of great variation-reduction meetings, then I'll show you one that crashed and burned. Next, I'll walk you through the practicalities of making a variation-reduction meeting happen—and work. Finally, I'll show you what's involved in creating and implementing a standard of care.

TWO PRODUCTIVE MEETINGS

When we began our variation-reduction project, the first specialty group I worked with was the Ear, Nose, and Throat Department. When we pulled the data on our five ENT physicians, it was clear that the illness they treated most often was chronic sinusitis, an inflammation/infection of the sinuses in the head. Variation in overall cost of the treatment of chronic sinusitis was determined mainly by the number of times per patient that a physician performed a flexible fiber-optic endoscopy—a procedure that provides rather spectacular views of the inside of the nose, the back of the throat, and the vocal chords, but costs much more than the traditional procedure of examining the throat and nose with a mirror.

After gathering and analyzing the data, we invited the ENT physicians to a variation-reduction meeting. The meeting couldn't have gone better. To start with, the physicians all attended, which I didn't deeply appreciate at the time, but which was, in retrospect, one of our really important early wins: getting all of a department's physicians in the same room at the same time is a crucial part of the variation-reduction process.

Second, the ENT physicians accepted the data I showed them and immediately understood its implications. When I asked them the one simple question—"Why do you think there's such a variation?"—there was an uneasy silence. This group did not have any senior physicians to take the lead; they were all about the same age. No one knew how to respond. One finally spoke up and said, "You know, I'm embarrassed by this, because I thought that I was doing the same thing as all of my colleagues; I'm surprised to find that there's such a big variation here." His colleagues piled on in agreement.

This was my first experience watching the kind of realization I was later to see repeated in specialty group after specialty group, especially when discussing the most common ailments that the specialty treats. While it's very typical for physicians to discuss unusual cases with their colleagues and ask for advice, they very rarely talk about the common issues they deal with every day. After all, didn't they learn the treatment of common problems during training? Those problems aren't very interesting, so why discuss them? But when they consider the volume of these common treatment encounters and the variation in their treatment of them, suddenly the uninteresting becomes very interesting indeed.

Like many other specialties to follow, these ENT physicians had never seen data like this. It had never occurred to them that chronic sinusitis accounted for the majority of the cost for caring for their department's patients. Now, faced with the evidence of their variation in its treatment, they became volubly engaged in the kind of conversation that a variation-reduction team wants to hear. "Well," one of the physicians concluded enthusiastically, "We can create a standard and probably reduce the overall cost."

The same realization can also occur with physicians less willing to accept the data at face value. For example, when we sat down to talk with our Neurologists about their variation in the use of MRIs in the workup of a headache, they looked at the variation and grumbled, "I can't believe this data."

One of the Neurologists sat up straight in his chair and declared, "I can't believe that there is a Neurologist within 100 miles of where I'm sitting who wouldn't get an MRI on a new patient with a headache."

And the guy sitting right next to him said, "I don't do that."

And the first guy said, "Really? Well, when do you get it?"

"Well, I get it under these circumstances."

"Well, *I* get it under *these* circumstances."

Others soon joined in, and it was the start of a standard for the use of MRI in the workup of a headache. These two Neurologists with offices right next to one another had developed startlingly different practice patterns. And because both of them thought that their colleagues all acted as they did, they had never asked each other the question. Without the variation-reduction meeting, the discussion would never have taken place.

THE MEETING FROM HELL

I hope you have the same kind of early successes with your variation-reduction meetings that we had with ours, but some of our successes were sheer luck. If your luck runs the other way, the long-term effects could be devastating.

We had a bad experience with our Rheumatologists, who practice in a geographically dispersed area. (Luckily, our project was already pretty well established by the time of this encounter, so while the episode was distressing, it did not devastate the project.) We had tried several times to schedule a Rheumatology variation-reduction meeting, but never could get the Rheumatologists together in person because of scheduling and travel issues. So for a first meeting, we decided to try to gather as many of the Rheumatologists as we could in person and connect with the others by phone, using WebEx technology to display our graphs and PowerPoint presentation. As it turned out, though, the only people who showed up in person were the variation-reduction team members. All the Rheumatologists were on the phone. The variation-reduction champion who was leading the meeting was at a severe disadvantage: she didn't know the Rheumatology Department's politics, hadn't met some of the physicians, and couldn't recognize the physicians on the phone by their voices. When she began with our usual preliminary remarks about why PAMF needs to reduce variation, one of the Rheumatologists jumped in, saying that he just didn't think the project was necessary and that all we would accomplish was reducing our revenue. The variation-reduction team members gave what we thought was a reasoned response to this type of objection, but our rationale clearly did not satisfy him.

At this point, we should have slowed down to directly engage with the physician's objections, but we moved on to the next step, displaying a sample variation-reduction graph for Rheumatology. As the physicians began to find themselves on the bar chart (where each bar represented the practice pattern of one Rheumatologist, identified by name), it became clear to all that the physician with the most initial distrust of the variation-reduction program was also the physician with the highest per-patient charges. Immediately, he began sparring over the phone with the physician with the lowest per-patient charges. These two physicians had philosophies of practice that were quite different. While they didn't know one another very well, they had a history of disagreements, and the fact that they weren't in the same room made it easier for them to take verbal jabs at one another.

Communication at a distance, whether by phone, E-mail, or Internet, disinhibits some people, allowing them to act in ways that they would never do if communicating face to face. Not understanding the history of volatility between these two physicians, the variation-reduction champion added some of her own verbal mistakes and the whole thing degenerated into a disastrous meeting that went nowhere fast.

It took us months to restore calm among the Rheumatologists, because everybody was mad at everybody else. One of the Rheumatologists absolutely refused to participate any further, and we had to replace him on the Rheumatology variation-reduction team. (Work on variation reduction is voluntary at PAMF and we have no penalties for non-participation. Fortunately the vast majority of our physicians find this work worthwhile.) Despite our apologies, our attempts at service recovery, and our decision to change the staff used to facilitate the meetings, negative feelings about variation reduction continued among the Rheumatologists for more than a year. Eventually, the reconstituted variation-reduction team was able to assist the Rheumatology physicians to establish several standards for the treatment of rheumatoid arthritis that were accepted by all, even the contrarian. But it took a long time.

This type of disaster can have widespread implications. It's difficult enough to get physicians to begin to participate in variation reduction in the first place; when they hear from a colleague how badly a meeting went, the degree of difficulty skyrockets. (It's curious how one bad meeting never seems to die, while people quickly forget all the meetings that ended with physicians saying, "This was really worthwhile.")

So let me give you a few tips on handling your variation-reduction meetings: how to set up the right-sized meeting, make it actually happen, run it, adapt to the needs of the meeting's participants, and foster productive synergies among colleagues.

SET UP THE RIGHT-SIZED MEETING

Getting the right-sized variation-reduction meeting is important. You can't have a good discussion with only one or two physicians in the room; three or four is usually the minimum number needed to have a collaborative process and successful dialogue.

Small- and medium-sized departments offer the advantage of having direct democracy; everyone in the department can participate. Our first meeting with the five ENT physicians went well, as did our first meeting with Oncology, attended by all 12 Oncologists. Having everyone in the department at each of those meetings made for an outstanding experience; the engagement was palpable.

However, when we started working with departments beyond about 10 to 15 physicians, we began to have problems. A few people would dominate the conversation while others would sit back and say nothing. We made it part of the variation-reduction champions' meeting plan to track who had spoken up and who had not and to specifically ask for input from those who were quiet. This was particularly important when some of the attendees were calling in to the meeting because it was easy for those "call-in" physicians to take a very passive role. The champions were instructed to periodically ask those on the phone what they were thinking.

In even larger departments such as Primary Care or OB/GYN, it just wasn't practical to invite everyone in the department to the meeting. So who to invite? In general, we invited one or more physicians from each of our four clinical sites, asking them to discuss possible variation-reduction topics with their colleagues before coming to the meeting. We wanted them to express their own views and represent the aggregated view of their clinical sites.

When we realized that few of the "representatives" had actually consulted their colleagues in advance of the meeting, we were dismayed; their opinions were just their opinions. But physicians need data in front of them before they can start a discussion on standard setting. No data, no discussion. And we noticed that not having discussed possible topics with their colleagues didn't seem to inhibit the representatives' process anyway. The same types of discussions occur in large department meetings as in small department meetings in which all members are present; the difference is the work needed afterwards to spread the result of the large department meeting to those who were not present.

When it's time for you to invite physicians to your first variation-reduction meeting, make sure to "right-size" the meetings. The larger the number of participants, the harder it will be to schedule the meeting. Trying to schedule an initial meeting with more than 6 attendees becomes difficult because of on-call schedules and other commitments. A department of as many as 60 can be represented by 6 physicians.

Geography is an important consideration. Try to include representatives from each of the clinical locations in your system. If you have three Dermatology offices, for example, make sure that at least one representative is present from each of the three offices. If you have the opportunity, it's also a good idea to invite physicians who represent both those new to the practice and those who have been in practice for some time. It's also very useful to have a "thought leader," a physician with stature who is very well-respected by others in the group.

MAKE THE MEETING HAPPEN

Getting physicians to actually *attend* a variation-reduction meeting is one of the key sticking points in the whole process. You'll have a number of hurdles to overcome. First, there will be some degree of skepticism on the part of the physicians. You'll find yourself fielding comments such as, "What is this all about?" and "Are we going to get yelled at?" But a more mundane hurdle is the logistical difficulty of getting the people in the same room at the same time. The two most distant of PAMF's four clinical sites are more than 40 miles apart. Now add the fact that most meetings are held after office hours, which means driving during rush-hour traffic. When faced with a 30- to 60-minute drive at the end of a long day, some physicians will just say, "I'm not coming." So we had to come up with a number of different strategies that we thought might help get people together.

We had originally thought that distance technology—phone or video-conferencing and WebEx presentations—might be one way of doing things; we found instead that technology, as an alternative to getting people in the same room at the same time, was a poor second choice. We decided that it made no difference how good the technology was. It's too easy to do something else while on a phone conference and not pay the proper attention that variation-reduction discussions need. In addition, it's too easy to show a lack of respect. With in-person meetings, we've never seen contentious behavior. When people get together, there's much more of a conciliatory camaraderie-type vibe to the meeting.

(This is not to say that we never do phone conferences. We have found that conference calls can work for a second or third meeting, after the variation-reduction specialty team has already met in person. Participants can, for example, sort out the standard on the phone, but this only works after there's been some prior teambuilding at an in-person event.)

So how can you entice physicians to attend? The first strategy is obvious: you lure them with data. A little data sent out before the meeting will make them want to come to find out more. Our variation-reduction team always comes prepared with the data that the physicians have requested even if we don't think it's important. Whatever the physicians want, we try to make happen.

The next big issue is food. While you might get physicians to come to a first meeting without feeding them, they won't come back a second time. In the beginning, we let physicians pick restaurants at which to host the meetings, but that got to be a bit pricey, the environment could be noisy, and the physicians were often concerned that the discussion could be overheard. Our in-house catering service does a reasonable job of providing food for most meetings. Now we take physician groups to restaurants as a reward after they have gelled and become productive.

In addition to providing them with food, we do pay physicians an hourly rate (including drive time) to come to the meetings. It's not as much as they would make seeing patients, but it's enough that it means something to them, and it shows them that we value their time.

If variation reduction is to work, you have to get the physicians engaged. Data, food, compensation: whatever works. (This is where it can pay to have a resourceful administrative assistant.) At one point, one of our variation-reduction physician champions was having a tough time getting the Neurosurgeons together. He went so far as to offer to drive over to one physician's office, which was 30 miles from his own office, to pick him so he could come to the meeting. The Neurosurgeon declined the ride but did show up at the meeting. Persistence pays off!

STRUCTURE THE MEETING

When you get physicians in the room for a variation-reduction meeting, the first thing you need to do is convince them that the process is really necessary. You'll need to do this each and every time you meet with a new set of physicians. Reminding them why the organization needs to carry out variation reduction is crucial in engaging them to commit to the process.

At PAMF, we begin a typical first variation-reduction meeting by stating the problem: that until we began this initiative, we were pricing ourselves out of the market. By mid-2008, the economy—even in the robust Silicon Valley, where the Palo Alto Medical Foundation lives—was in the toilet. Unemployment was above 10%, and many patients were losing their health insurance because they had been laid off. Patients who still had insurance couldn't afford the procedures physicians were recommending because their high-deductible health insurance plans had saddled them with high out-of-pocket expenses. And everyone was being bombarded with information about how unaffordable healthcare was becoming and the uncertainties of healthcare reform.

This trifecta of external forces made it easier for our physicians to contemplate the changes necessary to make variation reduction successful. And these external forces are still present in our area today, although the economy has improved. As we approach the 2014 implementation of the

Affordable Care Act, the media coverage will increase. In a recent news conference, Peter Lee, the executive director of Covered California (California's health insurance exchange) said that people can expect the airwaves to start buzzing with an advertising campaign to inform people about the new insurance marketplace.[34]

But I think the case for variation reduction can be made even without such external pressures. As the second step of our initial variation-reduction presentation, we always share information about warranted and unwarranted variation and the history of variation reduction—in effect, part I of this book. We want to make sure physicians understand that variation reduction is not just some fad that we have concocted ourselves; rather, a need for it has long been established in the medical literature.

Those first few minutes of the meeting are the time to make a compelling argument for why you're asking the physicians to go through the variation-reduction process. We found out the hard way that we always needed to make our case before providing the physicians with their department's personally identifiable data. The moment you give the physicians the data, you lose them for all other purposes. First, all eyes scan to find their own names on the variation spectrum. Then, all minds strain to poke holes in the data they find objectionable.

I remember one of our early meetings with the General Surgeons, when I handed out two data sets to the physicians before we started the meeting. One set showed the charges for repair of inguinal hernia; the other showed charges for the removal of gallbladders. All heads went down as the surgeons burrowed deep into the data. One of my favorite surgeons, the one I'd let operate on me, found himself at the high end of the hernia cost data and said that he just couldn't understand it. He was sure that he was doing the procedure in the most cost-effective way. "I just don't believe this," he muttered. Then he turned to the next page, where he found himself to be one of the lowest-cost surgeons for gallbladder removal. Almost immediately, he said, "Now this is data I can believe in."

And in fact, he was right in both cases. There was an error in the hernia data set and this surgeon helped us understand how we needed to correct it. Learning from that meeting, we began to show data sets to the department's chief or one of its thought leaders before the initial variation-reduction meeting. This practice allows us to spot some of the obvious mistakes.

In the case of the General Surgeons, the mistake was that fees for the facility were added into costs for some surgeons, but not others. So we had to eliminate all the facility fees for everybody so we could compare one physician to another fairly. Unbalanced comparisons are a particularly common problem for large groups, where some physicians practice totally within the system so that all data is captured, while others sometimes work in settings where it is not possible to capture the data.

The next part of the first variation-reduction meeting is perhaps the most crucial. We ask the physicians the following question: Why does the variation exist?

The most common response is that the data are wrong; the data must have been collected improperly and analyzed incorrectly. We then begin to work through the objections, always taking the one-down approach, always welcoming correction. Eventually an opening occurs when we can ask the physicians what they do in a given situation. When one answers one way, someone else will answer differently. At this point, the data we used to frame the initial query are forgotten and the clinical discussion begins. The variation-reduction champion guides that discussion, taking notes and working toward consensus. Ideally, the meeting ends with a standard. If not, the variation-reduction champion summarizes the meeting in an E-mail and continues to try to reach consensus by E-mail interchanges or, if necessary, additional meetings.

ADAPT TO PARTICIPANTS' NEEDS

We discovered in our first variation-reduction meeting with Orthopedics that it was extremely important to be ready to adapt our agenda to participants' needs. That first meeting was actually almost comical. Independent and surgical in nature, Orthopedists are always a difficult group of physicians to work with. PAMF has basically two kinds of Orthopedists: the first are general Orthopedists who handle all types of orthopedic problems, including major joint replacements that most commonly result from degenerative disease; they treat patients who are older and who require hospitalization for the procedure. The other Orthopedists are sports medicine physicians who perform a lot of arthroscopy; they treat a younger, fit group of patients who generally have outpatient procedures. The joint replacement subspecialty has 42 physicians and mid-levels; the sports medicine subspecialty has 21.

Although we invited representatives from both subspecialties to the first Orthopedics variation-reduction meeting, only the sports medicine physicians showed up. Not particularly enthused with the idea of variation reduction, they wanted to pick a topic for the Orthopedics variation-reduction project that would affect only the joint replacement surgeons. Politely pushing back, we eventually got them talking about variation in knee arthroscopy—a much more appropriate subject for sports medicine.

The next Orthopedics meeting was equally unexpected, but for a different reason. By now we realized that we would have to split the sports medicine physicians and the joint replacement physicians into two separate projects. For this second meeting, we invited only the joint replacement physicians, the doctors who principally perform total-joint replacements for hips and knees—and who hadn't showed up for the first meeting.

We lost control of the conversation right away. For about the first hour, the Orthopedists delivered a harangue about all the problems they were facing with Stanford University Hospital, where they did many of their procedures. They had identified the variation-reduction team as "administration," and they wanted administration to fix the problems that they had been suffering for all these years. Blindsided, but following our one-down precepts, we didn't try to wrest the conversation back to our agenda; instead, we listened to theirs.

During this conversation, we learned that the Orthopedists had split into two subgroups whose members were at each other's throats. These subgroups differed in the way they coded their surgeries. Each subgroup was adamant that what it was doing was right, and what the other guys were doing was wrong. Physicians in the one subgroup said that every time they saw a patient, they used an ICD-9 code in the 800 series (acute injuries). The other group, equally adamant, said that they used 700-series codes (chronic injuries). Neither faction could be enticed to speak about variation reduction with such an abyss between them. Eventually, they agreed to let us bring in a coding expert to adjudicate the correct way to code their procedures. This issue could have been an insolvable problem: in the field of medical coding, even expert certified coders agree among themselves only 75% of the time. Fortunately, though, the coders were able to straighten out the issue: all the joint replacement Orthopedists now code the same way . . . at least for now.

Only after we engaged with the physicians on their own terms were they willing to put aside their agendas and begin to talk about the issue of variation reduction in Orthopedics. As you conduct your initial meetings, you, too, may encounter seething issues that prevent meaningful dialogue about variation. While it may seem as though it takes a long time to get down to the issue you want to discuss, you'll find that time spent listening to the physicians and gaining their trust is time well-spent.

FOSTER SYNERGIES

For the most part, we've found that it's unproductive to bring two specialty groups together for one variation-reduction meeting. But there are circumstances for which we do exactly that. When a specialty wants to do a variation-reduction project that includes imaging procedures, for example, we think it's a good idea to have Radiologists in the room when we discuss the project.

The first time the Pulmonologists met to discuss the issue of using CT scans to follow up on pulmonary nodules, no Radiologist was at the table. The Pulmonologists created what they thought was an appropriate standard and they set the standard in place. When the variation-reduction team pulled data several months later, we had to report to the Pulmonologists that essentially, there had been no change in their practice pattern.

When we examined the data we realized that two things were happening. First, PAMF Radiologists have the discretion to change the orders of a referring physician if they believe that the procedure isn't appropriate for the patient's clinical situation. And indeed, we found that on occasion, the Radiologists were changing orders from those that conformed to the Pulmonologists' new standard. Second, most of the CT scans performed had been ordered by Primary Care, rather than by a Pulmonologist. And while the Pulmonologists had developed and spread their standard among themselves, they had not formally spread it to Primary Care.

The second meeting, which included both Pulmonologists and Radiologists, was much more effective. Both specialties were concerned that patients receive no more radiation than is necessary to get the information. They agreed on a length of time between the initial scan and follow-up scans. They discussed when it was appropriate to do a full CT scan in follow up and when a limited CT scan would do. They went so far as to actually devise a protocol *during that meeting*, stating exactly how each scan would be performed. This was a first in our experience: developing and implementing a standard in a single meeting. By the next day, a new procedure for the Radiology technicians was put into place at all of our imaging sites. Subsequent data pulls showed an increase in the limited CT scans, reducing not only costs but the amount of radiation that patients must bear.

WRITE A STANDARD OF CARE

Most initial variation-reduction meetings don't result in the immediate creation of a standard of care. Participants need to think about the issue and find out what their colleagues and their specialty societies have to say about it. They want to go to the literature and find out if an evidence-based standard exists on indications for the procedure and how often to do it.

Over time, it has become a task of the variation-reduction team to prod physicians to actually write the standard and make sure everyone on the project team has a copy of it. It often takes a number of nudges. Typically, the specialists agree in a meeting on the standard but no one is willing to write it down. And so, a member of the variation-reduction team writes up a draft of the standard based on what's said at the meeting, and then sends the draft by E-mail for comment. The resulting E-mail thread clarifies and solidifies the standard.

Our first experience with creating a standard involved the five ENT physicians, who put the standard together and distributed it among themselves. After eight months, we analyzed their practice patterns. The data showed a clear difference between what they had done before the standard and what they had done after the standard had been put in place. All the physicians reduced their cost for the treatment of chronic sinusitis. All reduced the number of times they performed nasal endoscopy on patients with chronic sinusitis. Even the physicians who initially had low utilization of fiber-optic endoscopy found that when they used the standard that they themselves had created, they performed fewer procedures. The physicians on the high side dropped more than the physicians in the middle, who dropped more than the physicians on the low side, but everybody dropped.

According to our statistician, the ENT specialists decreased the mean, but the coefficient of variation remained the same. In other words, while they performed fewer procedures overall, variation was still there. That makes sense, because any clinical situation can combine both warranted and unwarranted variation: warranted variation is properly caused by differences among patients; unwarranted variation is caused by patient and physician preference, not medical necessity. When you successfully eliminate unwarranted variation among procedures, the volume of procedures decreases and the variation that remains is mostly of the warranted kind.

Although we did not know it at the time, reducing the mean while maintaining the coefficient of variation was a statistical change we were to see frequently in specialties that participated in the variation-reduction project. Creating a standard allows physicians to provide more appropriate care. Even physicians who are already doing appropriate care can improve.

SPREAD THE STANDARD

In small departments, the physicians who put together the standard are the same physicians who will implement it. In this case, there's no difference between creating the standard and spreading it. But in large departments, or in departments with interdependencies, spreading the standard is an essential additional step. When the Pulmonologists created their first standard, for example, no one notified the Radiologists or Primary Care Physicians and the standard had no effect. On our second attempt, the Radiologists and Pulmonologists worked together with the variation-reduction team to make the new standard known to the Primary Care Physicians. We used E-mails, posts to our physician blog, and an article in our physician newsletter to get the word out.

Our ad hoc efforts to publicize the Pulmonology/Radiology standard to the Primary Care Physicians were a great success. We decreased the number of unnecessary full CT scans and reduced the radiation exposure for many patients. Our key participants were few in number, highly motivated, and acting with the benefit of hindsight from the earlier failed effort.

But the variation-reduction team's experience with the Dermatology Department taught us that we needed to create a formal spread mechanism for departments' variation data and standards of care. Dermatology is a large department, with 30 physicians at four different clinics. It really was not possible to bring all the physicians together for a meeting, so we asked each site to send one representative to an initial variation-reduction meeting. With five representatives in the room—one from each region plus the Dermatologist who specialized in pathology—we showed several data sets.

The first data set was on variation in the treatment of acne. I thought this was an absolutely fascinating topic, because I was surprised to see so much variation in the treatment of this very common problem. But the Dermatologists took one look at it and said, "Ugh! Acne! We have to deal with acne all day long. We don't want to even think about this. Let's talk about skin cancers." I took a deep breath, remembered our principle of letting the specialists choose their own topics and said, "Fine, let's work on skin cancers." (In my heart, I really wanted them to work on the acne issue, and subsequently the Dermatologists did come back to it after they had gained experience working with the variation-reduction process. I believe that they came back to the acne issue in part because we did not force them to do it in the first round. Variation reduction was new to these specialists and they needed to experience it under their own terms.)

The meeting of the Dermatology representatives was active and engaging, and variation-reduction team members who participated left the meeting thinking that it had been very successful. Subsequently, we were copied on multiple E-mails through which the Dermatologists hammered out a standard for the treatment of basal-cell skin cancers. After several weeks, they had written a standard and told us that it had been a very successful process. We eagerly awaited the second round of data to see the effect of the new standard.

Six months went by; we did a second data pull and saw that the standard had had absolutely no effect. Disheartened, we wondered why this very engaged team of physicians had failed to make any significant change in their overall practice of the treatment of skin cancers. We decided to survey all 30 Dermatologists and were surprised to find comments in the survey such as "I thought the standard was a secret." It became clear that the Dermatology variation-reduction representatives had not spread the standard to their colleagues. We had assumed that they would go to their department's meetings and show the data and the standard they created from it. In fact, they had done neither. When we asked why, they told us that they felt uncomfortable discussing the variation data. They thought that by showing their colleagues the evidence of personally identifiable variation they were in some way criticizing them, and they were uncomfortable doing that. Without the context provided by the variation data, they'd found the standard hard to promote, so. . . .

From these discussions the variation-reduction team realized that it would be better for us to show the data to physicians in all the departments, first because we understood how the data was gathered and could answer those type of questions, and second because we were well-versed in a nonjudgmental method of presentation.

We also realized that it was our responsibility to make sure each standard was spread. We began with Dermatology, coordinating with the representatives, and going to the individual clinic meetings, to show both the data and the standard. After we used this spread methodology, the third data pull for the Dermatologists (six months later) showed a significant decrease in the variation—and charges—for treatment of basal-cell carcinomas.

We found the same structural issues in OB/GYN, another very large department. We have 75 physicians and mid-levels in the OB/GYN Department; when the representatives met, it was a very engaged group whose members responded to the variation data sets and created a standard of care. Again, though, they were very uncomfortable going back to their colleagues to present the variation data and thus the standard. We attended each local OB/GYN Department meeting to help the representatives spread the standard, and we made that our own standard procedure.

It's common to talk about organizing physicians as "herding cats": we're famously strong-willed and independent. But throughout our variation-reduction project, we've found that we can herd physicians with the cream of data and a safe place to purr.

CHAPTER 15

Solving Problems

Running a variation-reduction program is very rewarding. It's personally rewarding because you can see the impact of your work in increasing value to your patients. It's organizationally rewarding because it improves your ability to contract with health plans and employers and helps you improve access for your patients.

However, variation reduction is not always a bed of roses. You will certainly encounter your share of difficulties as you implement your project, as did we. I hope the examples I share here of problems and solutions at PAMF will give you ideas about how to overcome problems of your own.

Looking back, I see that most of our difficulties were caused by one or the other of two things: people issues and data issues. Some of our most difficult problems were caused by thinking that we faced one type of issue when we actually faced the other—or didn't realize that we were facing both at the same time. And the master solution to all of them was training and supporting variation-reduction champions.

GETTING TO THE HEART OF THE MATTER

Some issues you'll encounter are strictly people problems. As there is variation in practice patterns among specialists, there is variation among the specialties with regards to adopting the variation-reduction process. In general, the surgical specialties seem to embrace this process more easily than the medical specialties. When our plastic surgeons met to review their variation data, for example, the conversation was truly exciting. They quickly realized that their use of an assistant surgeon was the main difference in their variation, and the discussion between the surgeons who used an assistant and those who didn't was a learning experience for everyone.

On the other hand, the meetings with the Cardiologists were much more difficult. After an initial meeting that consisted mostly of arguing about the data, they turned the whole problem over to one of their colleagues who had experience doing clinical research. He wanted us to turn over all our raw data so he could do his own analysis. So we did.

Several weeks went by. Eventually I gave him a call.

"What's happening?" I asked.

"Oh. You're right," he said. "There really is variation here. I did these statistical tests to confirm it, and you're absolutely right! I've sent this information to all the other Cardiologists, and we're in the process of creating a standard."

One would like to say this is the end of the story and that the Cardiologists all agreed from that point on to participate actively in the variation-reduction project, but the reality was that it was only that one Cardiologist who was convinced. The rest of his colleagues remained significantly opposed to the idea.

In a situation like this, persistence by the variation-reduction champions is key. We persisted in contacting the Cardiologists on a regular basis, asking them what type of data they wanted us to get for them and asking to set up follow-up meetings. After many rebuffs we finally brought out the big guns: we took the Cardiologists' opposition to senior leadership. Members of leadership had assured the variation-reduction team that they were willing to help, but we had held off contacting them, believing that we needed to exhaust all of our resources before escalating the issue. Only with a strong case for non-compliance would we turn to the leadership.

With the intervention of our senior leadership, the Cardiologists did move off the rock of "We don't want to participate." At that time they were trying to get support from the organization to advance their work. Leadership told the Cardiologists that to be considered for these extras, they needed to participate in variation reduction.

What we learned was not to be afraid to bring in the boss when things are not moving. While we still adhere to the "work from the bottom up" rule, sometimes a nudge from the top is needed to break inertia. (More on the continuing saga of how we got the Cardiologists involved with variation reduction later in this chapter.)

Even with leadership buy-in, sometimes we still can't get physicians to the table. After we sorted out the schism issues with our Orthopedists, our sports-medicine physicians decided to tackle the issue of over-utilization of knee arthroscopy . . . but one key physician was missing from the meeting: the individual who did the most knee arthroscopies in the entire organization. He had, been invited to the meeting, of course, but he refused, saying that he never went to any of these types of organizational meetings. All he wanted to do was take care of his patients. Period. This Orthopedist was a well-known and widely respected expert in the treatment of knee problems; without his input, any knee arthroscopy standard would be suspect.

The variation-reduction team went to his department chair and had a long talk regarding our need for this physician's participation in the project. We left the meeting expecting movement: we had a commitment from the department chief to speak to the recalcitrant physician and a timetable for the discussion, and we fully expected that the intervention had worked. But what happened was just the opposite. The department chief felt very uncomfortable speaking to this physician and, in fact, never sought his cooperation to join the variation-reduction project.

So what do you do when this happens? We had already pushed it to leadership. We could have taken the issue to our board of directors, but to line up the power of the entire organization against a single physician—and for a voluntary project—seemed inappropriate. We decided that it would be better to just pick another topic and work on something that we could get results on. Some battles you just can't win, or the cost of winning the battle is too high. There was a lot more work to be done in Orthopedics and sports medicine, and, in fact, we did get several projects going in that department. Our hope is that we can come back to knee arthroscopy in the future and even persuade the recalcitrant physician to come to the meeting. It could happen.

Amusingly, another people-problem we've had is just the opposite of recalcitrance: departments that want to race ahead. Some physician groups get very excited about this type of work and want to take on projects that are too difficult, especially if they haven't had much experience in the variation-reduction process. To set these physicians up for success, we try to slow them down by setting up hurdles that they must overcome.

We ask them, "What's the first thing you'll need to know? And, after you know that, what's the second thing?" Asking them to think concretely about the necessary steps leads them to manage their project in a more realistic manner.

One of our very aggressive variation-reduction groups was Urgent Care. After their very first meeting, they wanted to move on to a second project. The variation-reduction team had to slow them down, to make sure that variation-reduction became a way of life, not just a meeting-by-meeting "one and done." So we set up a hurdle. We knew by now that spreading a standard is as important as creating the standard. The Urgent Care centers have a fair number of per-diem physicians, although the bulk of the shifts are handled by full-time physicians from PAMF. So we asked the Urgent Care variation-reduction group how they were going to spread the standard to the per-diem physicians. They eventually came up with a system whereby the standards were stored in the same place as the per-diem physicians' timesheets. All per-diem physicians had to sign off on the standards before they could sign off on their timesheets and get paid.

MINDING THE GAPS

Some issues you'll encounter mostly involve data problems. Although we don't promise or even seek perfect data sets, we must be confident that the data are complete enough to be useful and not to lead to erroneous conclusions. Using encounter or claims data does have some problems, so when you pull data for a particular entity, you'll have to go over them very carefully to make sure they aren't distorted.

First and foremost, you need to look for data gaps. For example, you're likely to find that your initial data pulls frequently leave out one or more physicians whom you know are doing the work in question. Sometimes your investigation is fairly straightforward: you can match the roster of the particular specialty with the data you have pulled and see if everybody's there. If data pulled from a department of a dozen Urologists show only nine, you know there's a gap in personnel. What's harder to spot is a gap in time. Data should appear for every specialist for every month. If they don't, you need to know why. We've seen initial gaps of as little as a month or two up to as much as several years. There's always a reason for a gap, but it may take a bit of detective work to find why the data are missing.

A good illustration of this issue involves our review of the treatment of prostate cancer. One of the treatments for prostate cancer is a drug called Lupron, which inhibits testosterone and therefore inhibits the growth of the cancer. PAMF has three different Urology clinics. When we first pulled the treatment data, it appeared that Urologists at two of the sites used Lupron on a regular basis, but the third site hardly used it at all. Given that we were actively looking for clinical variation, it would have been easy to assume that we had found it. But I put on my Sherlock Holmes deerstalker hat, visited the Urologists at the third clinic site, and asked, "Are you using this drug? It's a pretty standard treatment."

And they said, "Oh, yeah. We use it all the time."

So I started asking sequential questions, nailing down the workflow. "When you decide to use Lupron, how do you enter the order?" I asked.

The answer to that question was reasonable and led to the next question: "Do you give the injections in the office?" (Which is what physicians did at the other two sites.)

And they said, "Oh, no. We don't do that. We send the patients down to the cancer infusion center, and they give them the injections there." (Although the other two Urology clinics were also located near cancer infusion centers, they didn't use them for these injections.)

So I ambled down to the nearby cancer infusion center and said to the clerk, "What happens when one of the Urologists sends a patient down here for a Lupron injection?"

The clerk told me that she scheduled the patient for the injection.

"Well, when you do that," I asked, "which doctor do you list as the patient's doctor for this injection?"

And she said, "Well, since the Urologists aren't in this clinic, I always put down the name of the Oncologist who's in the infusion center that day, because if something goes wrong, the Oncologist is the first person I would call."

At that point I realized that, despite our focus on getting physicians to code things consistently, sometimes it's a person way down in the trenches who makes a decision that stymies data collection. When I went back to our data warehouse, I recoded those missing Lupron injections, filled the data gap, and was able to present to the Urologists their true variation.

The success of my Sherlock Holmes impersonation made a big impression on me, and I vowed to go to the source whenever the data we collected and analyzed didn't make sense, a practice that helped me understand another truly puzzling set of data.

Over time, the variation-reduction team has found that linking the use of a standard of care to physicians' clinical judgment is key to getting physicians to accept this process. When we speak with physicians, then, we always emphasize that a standard is something that physicians use to help guide their choices in caring for their patients, but that not every patient is served by adhering to the standard; use of a good standard is appropriate in only 80% to 90% of the patients, and its appropriate use depends on the patient's characteristics and the physician's clinical judgment.

We also encourage physicians to question the standards they create. If they find that a standard is not exactly correct, they should get together and change it. In that case, though, we ask them to do two things: first, make sure that all their colleagues know that they're changing the standard; and second, inform us, too, so we can monitor the situation. While the specialists are pretty good at the former, they sometimes aren't as good at the latter, which can lead to some interesting data conundrums.

As I discussed earlier, when the Allergists studied their diagnosis and treatment of allergic rhinitis, they discovered that their variation in the number of skin tests done during the initial evaluation (from as few as 20 to as many as 100) predicted the variation in the patient's annual cost. After research into the prevalence of local allergens, the Allergists set their standard for 40 skin tests.

When it came time to measure the effect of the standard, the variation-reduction team drew data on the number of patients who received exactly

40 skin tests during the initial evaluation of allergic rhinitis. We found virtually no one.

I was surprised, because this close-knit group of specialists had been eager to create the standard, and after the initial discussions there hadn't been much controversy about the number of skin tests to be used. So I went to one of the thought leaders in the allergy group and asked him why they weren't using their standard.

Perplexed, he said, "We *are* using the standard."

"But it doesn't seem that anybody is getting 40 skin tests. They're all getting more," I said.

"Oh. I forgot to tell you," he replied. "We changed it from 40 to 43 because we had forgotten about one group of common potential allergens in the community."

When we ran the data using 43 tests as our target, we found that more than 80% of the patients were being diagnosed using the standard.

We probably would have figured it out ourselves had we asked the analyst to create a graph showing the number of skin tests received per patient. Instead we had asked a more focused question: "How many patients exactly received 40 tests?" The analyst gave us the right answer; unfortunately, we had asked the wrong question. As I said: some "clear" data problems turn out to be people problems.

TURNING OVER THE STONE

After you understand the way people and data issues interact, you'll notice that many problems you encounter clearly involve both, especially when coding is involved; your physicians' agreement about which ICD-9 codes to use can mask or unmask true clinical variation.

One such problem was the general surgeons' project, which had to do with their most common procedure: using laparoscopy to remove gallbladders for gallstones. In laparoscopy, a surgeon inserts fiber-optic tools through the wall of the abdomen to remove the gallbladder without making a large incision. (It's truly an amazing improvement in technology: the open operative removal of a gallbladder used to involve at least a week's stay in the hospital, several weeks of recovery, and a major-league scar on the patient's belly. Now patients go home the same day; some surgeons even perform the procedure on an outpatient basis. Recovery time for the patient is also dramatically reduced. So this is quite an improvement over the old open procedure.)

I wasn't expecting anything dramatic from this project: I assumed that all the general surgeons were using this newer technique, and indeed they were. However, a small number of them were also performing a second procedure 80% of the time: an intra-operative cholangiogram (IOC), which allows a surgeon to visualize the common bile duct to confirm that no gallstones have been retained. Most of the frequent utilizers of IOC worked in one surgery clinic. All of them had been trained in the same surgery training program.

When I went to one of the surgeons who frequently did an IOC and asked my usual question, "Why do you do this?" he said that the procedure prevented postoperative complications, specifically that it reduced the risk of a retained gallstone, which could cause pancreatitis. When he was in training, he said, his chief wouldn't let him leave the operating room without doing an IOC. To this day, he said, as he neared the end of a gallbladder removal, he still heard in his head the voice of the chief saying,"It's time to do the IOC." Although it had occurred to him that it might be an unnecessary procedure in many cases, he found it hard to stop because all his immediate colleagues were doing the same thing.

I told this surgeon that reducing the risk of retained stones was obviously beneficial to patients, and if this procedure did what he thought it was doing, we should spread it to the other surgeons. So we decided to look at five years of gallbladder removals at PAMF and their subsequent complications. In general, the surgeons were coding this clinical situation with the ICD-9 code of 574, which is cholelithiasis (gallstones). When we examined surgical encounters with the 574 code, we found very few cases where postoperative complications were due to retained stones and no difference in their incidence whether or not a surgeon performed the IOC: a clear case of a "people" issue among the general surgeons.

Still, we wanted to make sure we didn't have a data gap, so we interviewed the general surgeons to better understand their workflow. In some cases, the surgeons involved Gastroenterologists before the procedure; in other cases, they were brought in during the postoperative period. (In part, this difference was due to the availability of Gastroenterologists with the skills needed to evaluate and treat a common bile duct obstruction.)

When we looked for Gastroenterology encounters with an ICD-9 code of 574, we found very few, which alerted us to data issues: we knew that the Gastroenterologists were seeing the patients because the surgeons told us they were, but we did not find them in the data when we filtered based on the 574 diagnosis. When we filtered by patient instead, we found that Gastroenterologists were using the ICD-9 code of 576 to code their encounters with the same patients. The 576 code is biliary obstruction. From the surgeons' point of view, the problem for the patient was the gallstones in the gallbladder; for the Gastroenterologist, the problem was an obstruction of the common bile duct. So the code assigned changed depending on whether the specialist was looking through a laparoscope or a GI endoscope.

Now in possession of complete data, we looked at the surgical complications again and still found no evidence that doing the IOC reduced the incidence of postoperative complication. Armed with this information, the surgeons established a standard of care detailing which clinical characteristics of a patient required the use of the IOC after a laparoscopy and which didn't. Although this process took almost a year to complete, during that year, the frequent utilizers decreased the number of times they did the IOC even before the standard was set in place. Just talking about the issue and raising everyone's awareness of the issue changed the surgeons' behavior.

About a year after the standard was adopted, I had the opportunity to speak again to the surgeon I'd originally interviewed. He told me that he still hears a voice in his head at the end of a laparoscopy—but it's no longer his old surgical chief. Now he hears *me* asking, "Why are you doing this?" I guess that's progress.

TRAINING VARIATION-REDUCTION CHAMPIONS

Understanding in advance the problems you'll face in a variation-reduction program allows you to create a process for resolving them—and sometimes heading them off before they begin. As the variation-reduction project at PAMF has matured, we've found that one of the most important parts of our work is recruiting and training great variation-reduction champions.

As I've already noted, the physicians we want to work with are the ones who are recognized by their peers as the doctors they themselves would want to see. For the PAMF program, we've had the privilege of attracting a number of respected clinicians who are enthusiastic about variation reduction. We've found that our most successful recruits are physicians who already come to us with experience in process improvement, energy for the challenge of the meetings, and exuberance in celebrating with their colleagues when a standard is set.

And then we train them.

The first step in our on-boarding process is to assign each new variation-reduction champion an experienced mentor who meets individually with the new champion at least once a week. The mentor goes over the basics of how to get data and organize them into a form that physicians can assimilate, how to run a variation-reduction meeting, and especially the idea of the "one-down" process.

The mentor also teaches the new champion to think of variation reduction as a campaign. Just as you would plan a political campaign or an advertising campaign, it's very important to think about variation reduction in terms of long-term change. This mindset is particularly true when you're trying to convince physicians to change their long-standing clinical practices.

Toward that end, the mentor explains the importance of the language we use. Words like "good" and "bad" or "outlier" are not in a champion's lexicon because they have negative connotations and they put physicians on the defensive. Because terms like "guidelines" and "best practices" evoke the failed managed care campaigns that tried to impose behavior change on physicians previously, we impress on the new champion the importance of the phrase "standard of care," the agreed-upon clinical practice that the physicians themselves set. The word "standard" seems to fit, and physicians are quite willing to accept it.

The mentor explains the need to tread softly when speaking about the financial aspects of variation reduction. We teach new champions to avoid phrases like "costs" or "revenue to the foundation" or "income to the physicians." Instead, we substitute the phrase—and idea—of "cost to the patient," or, increasingly, "value to the patient." Our physicians are acutely aware that with the increasing use of high-deductible health plans, many of our patients are having difficulty paying for healthcare. By speaking about cost or value *to the patient*, we focus the process of physician decision making on how decisions affect the whole patient and how physicians' participation in variation reduction helps their patients afford healthcare.

At the same time, as the new variation-reduction champions are learning the philosophy and terminology of variation reduction, they begin to experience the process in action. They attend our weekly staff meetings and, as much as possible, shadow veteran champions as they facilitate variation-reduction specialty meetings. They meet with data analysts to understand how data are gathered, analyzed, and visualized for presentation to the specialists.

One of the most valuable tools we have developed is a mock variation-reduction meeting, where the new champion plays the role of facilitator and the rest of the variation-reduction staff members play a variety of roles: the apathetic specialist, the specialist with a different agenda, the skeptical specialist, and other potentially difficult personality types we encounter during variation-reduction meetings. (Some also play cooperative, engaged specialists!) During these mock meetings, one member of the team functions as a coach who stays above the fray, calls time-outs for consultation, and takes notes so we can give accurate feedback to the new variation-reduction champion.

Holding mock variation-reduction meetings benefitted not only our new champions; it also forced us to create explicit standards for ourselves. Realizing that every good meeting has a predictable structure helped us ensure that a new facilitator would include all of its necessary parts.

In preparation for our mock variation-reduction meetings, we provide the new champion with sample variation data. This data set includes some hidden flaws (just like real data sets) so the champion will have to answer the objections of the physicians during the mock meeting. The champion works with an analyst to understand the data and prepare a presentation. The champion prepares a meeting agenda, which consists of three parts:

goals for the meeting, the rationale for variation reduction, and presentation and discussion of the data.

The new champion starts the mock meeting by making sure everyone knows everyone else, setting the ground rules for behavior, stating the variation-reduction team's goal for the meeting, and asking individual participants to express their own goals. This latter action is important, because it sets the expectation that everyone participates; the conversation will not be dominated by a few vocal members. It's the facilitator's responsibility to make sure we get everyone's oar in the water to move the process forward. The champion ends these preliminaries by reviewing the agenda.

Next, the champion provides participants with the rationale for variation reduction. In getting this chance to deliver and hone their presentations in a mock meeting, new variation-reduction champions often learn that they need to understand the variation-reduction rationale and process in more depth than they had thought. (This certainly is an example of the old saying that the best way to learn a subject is to teach it!)

The next part of the meeting is devoted to presenting the data. Here, the new variation-reduction facilitator learns to put into practice the open-ended, nonjudgmental questions that lead to illuminating clinical conversations. (The fun comes in for the other participants when we get to make the process difficult. It helps us work off some of our own frustrations!) Living through this experience helps the new champion learn how to not chase after the physicians. Like trying to capture a dog that has slipped its leash, physicians in these meetings slip away ever faster the more you run after them. Rather, the champion must stand still and simply ask, "Why does this variation occur?"

Learning how to wait and listen is key to facilitating an initial variation-reduction meeting. The variation-reduction champion facilitates the conversation and nudges it back towards variation when it starts to drift away. Sometimes the task is as easy as asking physicians, "So what goes through your mind when you're making the decision to consider ordering this test, doing this procedure, or prescribing this medication?"—inviting them to express their thought processes out loud.

Sometimes the task is considerably harder. Because it's important that everybody get on board, we train the new variation-reduction champion to engage in particular, those physicians who are most opposed to the entire process. A champion can't duck the tough questions, or people will draw the conclusion that the process isn't grounded in reality.

For example, most physicians know that a lumbar-spine MRI is of limited use in patients with new back pain. They also know that more and more patients come in demanding this expensive test anyway. So it's not uncommon during a variation-reduction meeting to hear a question such as, "How am I supposed to explain to the patient that this test isn't necessary?" In fact, this is a standard question that we throw at new champions; they need to have a ready answer. If the champion just turns to a physician and says, "Well, you just explain it," the physician isn't going to be very impressed . . . which is of no help.

Sooner or later, a variation-reduction champion is going to be flummoxed by a question, and we prepare them for that, too: we encourage the champion to ask the attendees, "Has anybody found a way to deal with this situation?" And usually, someone will have hit upon a strategy that works for them and that the other physicians can use also.

HELPING THE PHYSICIANS CHOOSE

As part of the initial variation-reduction meeting, physicians choose the project they want to tackle. I have said that "letting the physicians choose" is a basic tenet of variation reduction and a signal responsibility of the variation-reduction champion, and that's true, up to a point.

When I first met with the Obstetricians, early on in my initial variation-reduction project, I wanted to have them discuss C-section rates. Birth by C-section significantly increases the total cost of maternity care. In the United States, the C-section rate has risen from about 5% in the 1960s to more than 32% today, a national trend with many causal factors.[35] In our geographic area, once a woman delivers by C-section, subsequent delivering is routinely done by C-section, too, in order to avoid the possible catastrophic complication of uterine rupture. Data we developed at PAMF show significant variation among our OB/GYNs with regards to C-section rates, from less than 20% to as high as 45%. What we really need to know is an OB's primary C-section rate, but these data are difficult to obtain: some of the Obstetricians code so that we can distinguish between first-time and subsequent C-sections, but many don't. Even though PAMF has used very sophisticated electronic health records for 15 years, the OBs still do a lot of their documentation in paper "shadow" charts. Until we can separate primary from subsequent C-section rates, we can't distinguish between warranted and unwarranted variation.

When I walked into the first OB variation-reduction meeting and hinted that C-section rates might be a good place to start gathering and analyzing data, they looked at me as if I had the plague. They said, "That's such a controversial issue, and it depends so much on what the patient wants." They didn't want to touch that topic so I backed off.

After some discussion, they said they would be happy to look at postmenopausal bleeding, which they see on a regular basis in their practices. The American College of Obstetrics and Gynecology had recently put out a position paper on the workup of postmenopausal bleeding, so it was fairly easy for them to modify that recommendation for their particular patient population, come to an agreement on the specifics of their standard of care, and adopt the standard.

They were successful in this initial project, so the next time they had a meeting about developing a new standard they took on a more difficult topic: the frequency of performing Pap smears. With experience behind them, they were successful again.

At a recent variation-reduction meeting, one of the OB representatives suggested that maybe they're actually at a point where they can start looking at the variation data for C-section. It took time, but as they became more comfortable with the process, and as they experienced success in its implementation, they became willing to work up to addressing an extremely difficult topic. In the variation-reduction team's interactions with the obstetricians, our "campaign" has worked just the way it ought to: by letting the physicians choose.

To be clear, the goal is *not* to give physicians free rein; the goal is to provide the right amount of guidance to ensure that physicians embrace variation reduction and create projects with potential for success. Our champions don't abdicate responsibility for the work of variation reduction, and neither should yours.

When working with specialty groups that are resistant, for example, variation-reduction champions may need to be creative while keeping their eyes on the long-term goal. One way that specialty groups resist participation is by proposing projects that affect others rather than the specialty itself. I mentioned earlier how our first efforts with the Cardiologists required intervention from senior leadership. When we got the Cardiologists back for a second meeting, they said they had already come up with a project on their own: they would look at the screening rate for abdominal aortic aneurysms in male smokers over the age of 65.

The variation-reduction champion, a seasoned clinician, knew that this condition already has a non-controversial, Medicare-established standard, and it has a simple, noninvasive screening test that is typically ordered by Primary Care Physicians, not Cardiologists. When the champion mentioned these reasons not to address that topic, the Cardiologists said that they were quite willing to adopt the Medicare standard as it existed and that it would not be necessary to go through the motions of creating a local standard. Rather, the Cardiologists would remind their Primary Care colleagues about the Medicare standard; the variation-reduction team could follow on from there. The champion realized, of course, that the Cardiologists were creating a standard for the Primary Care physicians, who weren't involved in the discussion of the clinical problem or the "creation" of the standard.

Believing that they had fulfilled the requirement that each specialty participate in the variation-reduction process, the Cardiologists had started packing up their things and walking out of the meeting when the variation-reduction champion pulled them back in and re-opened the discussion.

"We said that we're usually looking for projects where evidence-based guidelines are absent and over-utilization is the issue," the variation-reduction champion reminded them mildly. "In this case, there's already an evidence-based guideline in place, and the variation seems to be due to under-utilization. Can we find a project that better fits the criteria for variation reduction?"

The Cardiologists said that the project they had proposed was the only project they were willing to undertake. Because of the difficulty of the situation, the variation-reduction champion decided to go ahead and work with the Cardiologists on that project, but insisted that the target group be the Cardiologists themselves: how often did a *Cardiologist* who saw an unscreened male smoker over the age of 65 neglect to order a screening ultrasound for an abdominal aortic aneurysm?

Because of the perseverance and flexibility of the trained champion, the Cardiologists finally had a project they could try. As it turned out, they did find variation in their compliance with the Medicare standard and they did change their behavior. Their first project led to increased screening rates; with time, we hope to see a decrease in resistance to the variation-reduction effort.

While it's best to let the physicians choose, remember that there's room for variation, even in the way variation reduction is done. No standard is correct for every situation; as with all matters in medicine, clinical judgment is always required.

INSISTING ON VALUE

Another way that specialty groups resist participation in variation reduction is by avoiding the question of affordability ("cost to the patient") and drifting toward the question of quality. Quality is, of course, a major component of value:

$$Value = \frac{Appropriateness \times Quality}{Cost\ to\ Patient}$$

While there's nothing wrong with discussing ways to improve quality, we train our variation-reduction champions to recognize that discussing only quality in a variation-reduction meeting typically is avoidance behavior.

To move the discussion back slowly from quality to affordability, our champions make no judgmental statements and ask no pointed questions. Instead, they gently but inexorably remind the physicians why they're in the room.

When our Gastroenterologists had their first variation-reduction meeting, we could tell that they were very uncomfortable discussing the variation. They had decided to look at the use of colonoscopy for colon cancer screening. This was an area the variation-reduction team was very interested in too, because there was significant variation in both the cost and frequency of this procedure at PAMF. In addition, colonoscopy is the number-one outpatient procedure we do, far exceeding any other medical or surgical procedure.

The GI variation-reduction group met and wanted to look at the time it took to do a colonoscopy. Apparently, it's well-established in the GI literature that the amount of time taken to remove the colonoscope is an indication of how complete the procedure has been. If you remove the colonoscope too quickly, there's a chance of missing a polyp, and finding polyps is the whole purpose of the procedure.

At the meeting, the Gastroenterologists became enmeshed in a discussion about how to time and record the colonoscope "withdrawal time." Mindful that groups need to work out their own agenda items before being able to concentrate on variation, the variation-reduction champion listened for a while, but finally had to remind the group that the purpose of the meeting was to deal with affordability issues, not quality issues.

The GI people had trouble moving away from the concept of quality measures to the concept of affordability measures. We worked with them during many meetings before we finally came to a way of looking at colonoscopy from the perspective of affordability.

Finally, the Gastroenterologists agreed to look at the interval between screening colonoscopies for patients at low risk for colon cancer. The national standard is that a screening colonoscopy should be done once every 10 years for patients at low risk. But in speaking with many of my Primary Care colleagues, I learned anecdotally that some of their patients were being screened at a 5-year interval and others at a 10-year interval. The GI group agreed that low-risk patients should be screened every 10 years; they also believed that they had little variation in compliance with that standard. We had no hard data on how often low-risk patients were screened, and we were not even sure how to obtain the data. I think the GI group agreed on this topic because they thought that either we couldn't measure compliance or that it would take many years for us to gather the data. I think they hoped that by choosing what they thought would be a long-term project, the variation-reduction team would leave them alone until we had data to report.

Until then, most of our data had come from our billing system, but there was no way for us to use billing data to answer the question of what length of time physicians were recommending between colonoscopies. Still, we suspected that these data were in our electronic medical records (EMRs), so we set forth to dig them out. We discovered that at the conclusion of each colonoscopy, the GI specialist had to enter into the electronic medical record (EMR) the date the group planned to do the next screening test so the system could send out reminders to patients that they were due for their tests. By using some rather clever programming developed by our data analyst, we were able to go into the EMRs and find out when patients' next colonoscopies were scheduled—not done, but scheduled. Because GI specialists perform so many of these procedures, it took the variation-reduction team less than three months to gather enough data to show the GI specialists that they were not following their own guideline that a patient at low risk should have a colonoscopy once every 10 years. In fact, we found about a three-fold variation in adhering to the 10-year recall standard: some of the GI doctors were scheduling 5-year follow-ups one-third of the time.

These data surprised the Gastroenterologists and spurred them to look more closely at their process. As they stepped through the process, they found that in some cases it was not the physician making the decision but the medical assistant. Physicians had told medical assistants to schedule patients at low risk for a return visit in 5 to 10 years, so the medical assistants assumed that 5 years was the most beneficial interval to recommend. Although clearing up that piece of communication eliminated quite a few of the early recalls, it also revealed that other instances were due to Gastroenterologists who were not following the standard themselves. Seeing their own data in comparison to their colleagues spurred the physicians on to adherence to the standard, and a second data set pulled three months later showed a marked decrease in variation.

With the Gastroenterologists, we had started with a group that wanted only to discuss quality; with persistence, we got them to look at affordability. So the screening colonoscopy project turned out to be a major improvement in both value and the total cost of care: physicians who were performing colonoscopies every 5 years on patients at low risk ended up doing twice as many screening colonoscopies as warranted. Because the waiting time for screening colonoscopy is significant, adhering to the 10-year standard permits PAMF to screen twice as many patients.

We presented these data in a meeting with some health plan and employer groups present. I don't think that the employer groups quite grasped the significance of this change at first—until one of the health-plan executives turned to the employers and said, "I don't think you understand how important this is." He continued, "I have never heard of a medical group saying that—without building more ambulatory surgery centers and colonoscopy suites, or buying more colonoscopes—they can screen twice as many patients with the same amount of resources. This is truly an innovative approach."

I was pleased to hear that kind of comment by a health-plan executive. With variation reduction, we want people to realize that we have a proven way to clearly change the way we provide medical care at significant quality and a lower total cost of care.

◆ ◆ ◆

In this chapter, I discussed the two most common types of problems faced when running a variation reduction program—people issues and data issues—and the common solution for them both: the leadership of effective variation-reduction champions.

I leave you with three common threads you should always think of when you and your champions need to solve a problem.

1. Be persistent. It takes time for physicians to come around to this new way of thinking about medical practice.
2. Go to the source and ask a lot of questions. The more you ask, the more information you will gather and the better the data you can bring to bear.
3. Be open to the presence of warranted variation and welcome the clinical judgment of your physicians.

Part I of this book explained how PAMF followed the path of variation reduction; Part II described what a physician, physician leader, or a physician group administrator needs to do to bring an organization to the same point. Part III has delved into the practice of variation reduction, showing what to do and how to do it. Variation reduction is not about crunching numbers, or implementing top-down control, or rationing care, or eliminating physicians' judgment; it's about a new and better way of practicing medicine.

Conclusion

As a result of the 2012 presidential and congressional elections, and despite efforts in the House of Representatives to repeal, defund, or dismantle Obamacare (37 bills passed as of this writing), it is certain that the Affordable Care Act (ACA) will change the way many Americans obtain health insurance. Starting in 2014, those previously uninsured will be able to obtain affordable insurance through state or federal insurance exchanges.

How many employers will drop health insurance for their employees is uncertain, and so is the number of people who will obtain health insurance from the exchanges. In about half the states, the governors and state legislatures have refused the additional Medicaid money offered and have refused to set up state-run health insurance exchanges. These states will rely instead on a federally sponsored health insurance exchange.

These continued political maneuverings have led some physicians once again to adopt a wait-and-see attitude. I believe this foot-dragging is shortsighted. Whether physicians like or dislike ACA, we need—at a minimum—to plan how to care for the previously uninsured patients who will crowd into our offices and clinics with new insurance cards in hand.

While reimbursement rates for physician services from these exchange health plans have not yet been announced as of this writing, it's anticipated that the best-case scenario is a Medicare-like fee schedule; more likely these rates will be somewhere between those for Medicare and Medicaid. For previously uninsured patients and the physicians who care for them, this will be a win-win situation: patients will have affordable insurance and physicians will treat patients they previously would never have seen and be reimbursed for care they previously would have written off.

For most physicians and physician groups, however, this deck holds two wild cards. The first is how many patients (and their families) currently on employer-sponsored plans will drop into the exchange health plans. Under ACA, all employers with more than 50 employees must provide health insurance or pay a $2,000 per-employee/per-year penalty. The reality is that most employers are paying about $15,745 per employee, per year in healthcare costs.[36] Two thousand dollars versus nearly $16,000? For some employers this may be an easy financial decision.

The second wild card is whether patients who are newly insured (on plans with relatively low reimbursement) will crowd out the reduced number of patients with employer-sponsored insurance (on plans with higher reimbursement) for the limited number of office slots. In Oregon and Massachusetts, previously uninsured patients who were given insurance used it. In particular, they used many preventive services.[37] This scenario could result in physicians seeing more patients, working harder, and being paid less—not a workable long-term solution.

While most physicians worry about how ACA may reduce individual reimbursements, they should also worry about how little ACA does to address how to control the cost of healthcare. The cost of care is—as it always has been—in the hands of physicians. I argue that even those physicians who are motivated solely by personal financial concerns should strongly desire to decrease costs and thereby lessen the likelihood of employers dropping their employees into the lower-reimbursement state insurance exchanges.

It's physicians who will need to convince employers that they should continue to provide health insurance, even if it costs more, because they can provide more valuable care. In a competitive labor market, where employees are a valuable commodity, it's easy to see how an employer might come down on the side of a higher-cost/more-value health plan that would give the employer a competitive advantage in recruiting and keeping good employees. Even in a less-competitive labor market, there's an efficiency rationale for employer-sponsored health plans: employees with such plans more likely have better access to care and may be seen sooner and at more convenient times than employees with the exchange programs. The decision to go with the lowest-cost healthcare needs to be made in light of how much value that low-cost care provides the employer.

In my recent discussions with both employers and health plans, I find that people are increasingly talking about not only cost, but value. This book has described the way for physicians to create more value in the care they provide to their patients. The tool to create more value is variation reduction.

In 2010, California became the first state to implement the ACA, creating the California Health Benefit Exchange (HBEX), the nation's first state-run marketplace for individuals to purchase affordable health insurance. In its final solicitation, HBEX required qualified health plans (QHPs) wanting to join the exchange to commit to improving the delivery of care:

> One of the values of the Exchange is to serve as a catalyst for the improvement of care, prevention and wellness and reducing costs. The Exchange wants QHP offerings that incorporate innovations in delivery system improvement, prevention and wellness and/or payment reform that will help foster these broad goals. These may include various models of patient-centered medical homes, targeted quality-improvement efforts, participation in community-wide prevention or efforts to increase reporting transparency to provide relevant healthcare comparisons and to increase member engagement in decisions about their course of care. QHP bids that incorporate innovative models, particularly those with demonstrated effectiveness and a track record of success, will be preferred.[38]

But like the federal ACA itself, California's HBEX, marketed as Covered California, appears to be on the same path as most health plans over the last 20 years in its ideas about what *will* improve the delivery of care: its four federally designated "metals" plans (platinum, gold, silver, and bronze) imply differences in value, but their major differences are in their co-pays and deductible levels—that is, in who will pay and how much. On average, a 40-year-old man will pay $321 per month for the silver coverage, a 24% decrease in the current rates for this type of health insurance.[39] And while the guiding principles of Covered California include a focus on "results," its metrics appear to measure value only by compliance with evidence-based standards.[40]

If the Covered California mission is to improve value for California consumers, will it accomplish that goal? I think it depends on your point of view. From the point of view of previously uninsured patients, Covered

California greatly increases value: when you start at nothing, anything positive looks great. But if you take the view of patients previously covered by an employer-sponsored plan, the value is less obvious, especially if patients' customary physicians are not available on their new Covered California plans.

It looks like the major way that the ACA proposes to decrease healthcare cost is to decrease reimbursement to physicians and other providers. But it's simplistic to think that decreasing reimbursement on its own will increase value to the patient. What happens if physicians decide en masse to limit participation in the exchange plans? Patients may have health insurance but limited access to care. This situation already occurs today with some physicians refusing to see patients insured by Medicaid. Will the positive effect of reduced costs outweigh the decrease in value from limited access?

In 2011, Medicare changed the process by which durable medical equipment (DME) is supplied to Medicare beneficiaries, instituting a competitive bidding process that in effect lowered by as much as 40% reimbursement for home oxygen and power wheelchairs, two common DME items. Medicare is a significant portion of any DME company's business. The decrease in Medicare's reimbursement rates has forced DME providers to cut back on services to patients who are insured by Medicare and patients who aren't.

In the past, for example, most DME companies delivered equipment to patients' homes. Now many DME companies are telling patients to come and pick it up themselves. In addition, many DME companies are no longer stocking infrequently used equipment that has for them a low profit margin: they say that they can no longer afford to provide equipment that they cannot reasonably expect to make money on. The inevitable consequence of this diminution of service is that some patients will no longer be able to be treated in their homes and instead will have to spend more time in hospitals or skilled nursing facilities. Even a single extra day in the hospital costs far more than any piece of DME equipment.

Both Medicare and the DME companies are acting appropriately. Medicare wants to use competitive bidding to reduce the occurrence of fraud in the dispensing of DME and reduce its staggering cost. (In 2009, the Government Accounting Office reported that Medicare spent $8.1 billion on DME.[41])

DME companies are doing what they can to produce an appropriate service and still make a profit. However, when a patient ends up staying in the hospital longer than medically necessary or must be re-admitted because the DME company did not refill a home oxygen tank, the overall cost of care to that patient goes up while its value goes down.

Ideally the concept of Accountable Care Organizations (ACOs) could help determine the value proposition for healthcare. Those entities (physicians and/or hospitals) accountable for the care of a group of Medicare beneficiaries could use tools such as variation reduction to set standards for increasing value, not just reducing cost.

As the reimbursement for an office visit decreases, will physicians see patients more often and perform more procedures than necessary? Will the exchange recreate the "Medicaid Mills" of the 1980s with quick visits to less-qualified physicians?[42] We know that unnecessary office visits occur right now. For example, PAMF experienced a three- to four-fold variation in the number of visits for hypertension before development of our hypertension standard. By creating and adhering to a standard, we removed 5000 visits per year while increasing the number of patients whose blood pressure is under control, raising value for those patients and opening access for others. What would be truly innovative is for the federal and state insurance exchanges to insist that variation reduction be part of the quality measures for their health plans.

Whether it's Covered California or any other health insurance plan, the centerpiece of health insurance needs to be value. It's no longer enough to rack up the usual quality metrics and say we're providing value to our patients. Physicians need to create standards for care and hold ourselves accountable to those standards. Those standards are best set through a variation-reduction process.

How will the system hold physicians accountable for adhering to a standard? It may be as simple having a penalty attached to reimbursements for care that doesn't follow the standard. (Obviously such a program would have to provide reimbursement in aggregate, because some variation is warranted and expected. No system should penalize physicians for taking on the care of patients who are very sick or difficult to diagnose.) Medicare has started such a program with hospitals, reducing payments to hospitals with high re-admission rates.

What I know will not work is just shifting financial risk for patient care from the health plan to physicians. We tried that in the 1980s and 1990s with Managed Care and it didn't work. Physicians didn't like it and neither did the patients. Much of the talk today about ACOs sounds very reminiscent to the discussions in the 1990s about HMOs.

◆ ◆ ◆

I wrote this book to convince physicians that we can make a difference; indeed, that we're the only ones who can. As Atul Gawande notes, "The most expensive piece of medical equipment, as the saying goes, is a doctor's pen."[43] Physicians have long wanted it both ways. We don't want to think about the costs of care, we argue passionately and in public; medical decisions should be made without the influence of who pays for the care or how much the care costs. Yet physicians often demand to be incentivized to provide any care at all. (Part of my job is to negotiate physician compensation with hospitals and other organizations, so I am acutely aware of what physicians expect.) Specialists demand to receive "on-call" pay from hospitals to be available for emergencies. Primary Care providers say that they need to be paid extra to respond to patients by phone or E-mail. And all physicians want to be compensated for the extra work caused by working with computerized healthcare records. So an outside observer might be forgiven to wonder cynically whether it's really medical ethics that makes physicians disregard cost to the patient and the healthcare system—or whether it's financial incentives that drive the care.

I don't think either ethics or incentives dominate most medical decisions. I think it's how those decisions are made.

In our current system, medical decisions default to individual physicians, which leaves too much up to idiosyncrasy and chance. We need to change that default to a collaboratively determined standard that takes into account all the factors of value, cost, outcomes, and appropriateness.

PAMF's variation-reduction program shows that physicians are willing to change their default from individual to collaborative decision making:

when physicians come to consensus on a standard, physicians will use that standard. PAMF has spent a lot of time and effort on this project and we are committed to spending a lot more. If you haven't started yet, you need to do so now. The time for "wait and see" has passed.

The physicians at the Palo Alto Medical Foundation have made a good start on reducing variation and increasing value for our patients. I hope this book will help you begin a variation-reduction program, too, so that my grandchildren—and yours—will live in a country sound in both economy and health.

ENDNOTES

1. Council of Economic Advisers, the Executive Office of the President. *"The Economic Case for Health Care Reform: Update."* Washington, DC: Council of Economic Advisers, June 2009, p.1.

2. For example, breast cancer survival rates and asthma mortality are about the same in the United States as in other industrial countries. See Squires, DA. *Explaining High Health Care Spending in the United States: An International Comparison of Supply, Utilization, Prices, and Quality.* New York: The Commonwealth Fund, May 2012.

3. *Congressional Budget Report.* November 2012, p. 38. http://cbo.gov/publication/43692.

4. Ibid p. 45.

5. A national survey in 1970 showed the overall tonsillectomy rate to be 3.7. Freeman, JL et al. Changes in age and sex specific tonsillectomy rates: United States 1970–1977. Am J Public Health. 1982; 72(5): 488-491.

6. Personal communication with the author, March 2010.

7. See Antman EM, et al. ACC/AHA guideline for the management of patients with ST-elevation myocardial infarction—executive summary: a report of the American College of Cardiology/American Heart Association Task Force on Practice Guidelines (Writing Committee to Revise the 1999 Guidelines for the Management of Patients With Acute Myocardial Infarction). *Circulation* 2004;110(5):588-636.

8. Wennberg JE Gittelsohn A. Small area variations in health care delivery: a population-based health information system can guide planning and regulatory decision-making. *Science.*1973;182(4117:1102-1108.

9. Baker N, Whittington JW, Resar RK, Griffin FA, Nolan KM. *Reducing Costs Through the Appropriate Use of Specialty Services.* IHI Innovation Series white paper. Cambridge, MA: Institute for Healthcare Improvement; 2010. www.IHI.org.

10. National Priorities Partnership. *National Priorities and Goals: Aligning Our Efforts to Transform America's Healthcare.* Washington, DC: National Quality Forum; 2008.

11. Fuchs VR. The doctor's dilemma: what is appropriate care? *N Engl J Med* 2011; 365: 585-587.

12. The Washington Times. Editorial: The return of the death panels. The Washington Times. August 20, 2012. http://www.washingtontimes.com/news/2012/aug/20/the-return-of-the-death-panels/#ixzz27tdqn6b3?

13. Porter ME.What is value in healthcare? *N Engl J Med.* 2010; 363:2477-2481, December 23, 2010DOI: 10.1056/NEJMp1011024.

14. Kaplan G. Transforming the Delivery of Health Care: Better, Faster, and More Affordable [PowerPoint]. Institute of Medicine, October 2007. http://www.iom.edu/~/media/Files/Activity%20Files/Quality/HealthCareQualForum/KaplanPresentation102307.pdf

15. Gawande A. The cost conundrum. *The New Yorker.* 2009;85(16):36-44

16. Smith M, Saunders R, Stuckhardt L et al, eds. abstract. *Best Care at Lower Cost: The Path to Continuously Learning Health Care in America.* Washington, DC: The National Academies Press; 2012.

17. Institute for Healthcare Improvement. Evolution of IHI. Available at http://www.ihi.org/about/Pages/History.aspx.

18. Institute for Healthcare Improvement. Overview. Available at http://www.ihi.org/offerings/VirtualPrograms/OnDemand/Squirrel/Pages/default.aspx.

19. Baker N. Whittington JW, Resar RK, Griffin FA, Nolan KM. *Reducing Costs Through the Appropriate Use of Specialty Services.* IHI Innovation Series white paper. Cambridge, Massachusetts: Institute for Healthcare Improvement; 2010. (Available on www.IHI.org.)

20. Institute for Healthcare Improvement. The Breakthrough Series: IHI's Collaborative Model for Achieving Breakthrough Improvement. IHI Innovation Series white paper. Boston: Institute for Healthcare Improvement; 2003. http://www.IHI.org

21. Resar R et al. Using a bundle approach to improve ventilator care processes and reduce ventilator-associated pneumonia. *Joint Commission Journal on Quality and Patient Safety.*2005;31(5): 243-248(6).

22. Rinke M et al. Implementation of a central line maintenance care bundle in hospitalized pediatric oncology patients. *Pediatrics.* 2012; 130(4): e996-e1004; published ahead of print September 3, 2012, doi:10.1542/peds.2012-0295.

23. For more information on lean management, see John Toussaint's book, *On the Mend: Revolutionizing Health Care to Save Lives and Transform the Industry.* Cambridge, MA: Lean Enterprise Institute;2010.

24. Brownlee S. Too Much Prevention: What Not to Do in the Primary Care Setting. Slide Presentation from the AHRQ 2009 Annual Conference (Text Version). Agency for Healthcare Research and Quality, Rockville, MD, December 2009 http://www.ahrq.gov/about/annualconf09/brownlee.htm

25. See The Cochrane Collaboration: http://www.cochrane.org/cochrane-reviews/about-cochrane-library

26. Moyer V. Screening for cervical cancer: U.S. Preventive Services Task Force recommendation statement. *Ann Intern Med*; 2012. 156(12):880-891.

27. The American College of Obstetricians and Gynecologists, The Pap Test, 2011.

28. Fahimi J, Herring A, Harries A, at al. Computed tomography use among children presenting to emergency departments with abdominal pain. Pediatrics.2012;130(5):e1069-e1075.

29. Bren L. Frances Oldham Kelsey: FDA medical reviewer leaves her mark on history. FDA Consum. 2001 Mar-Apr;35(2):24-9.

30. Fisch R, Weakland J, and Segal L. *The Tactics of Change.* San Franciso: Jossey-Bass; 1982:34-35, 140-149.

31. Dawson-Saunders B and Trapp RG. *Basic and Clinical Biostatistics.* Norwalk, CT:Appleton & Lange; 1990:52-54.

32. Patel M, Dehmer G, Hirshfeld J et al. ACCF/SCAI/STS/AATS/AHA/ASNC 2009 Appropriateness Criteria for Cardiovascular Computed Tomography Echocardiography, the Heart Failure Society of America, and the Society of American Society of Nuclear Cardiology Endorsed by the American Society of Association for Thoracic Surgery, American Heart Association, and the Angiography and Interventions, Society of Thoracic Surgeons, American Foundation Appropriateness Criteria Task Force, Society for Cardiovascular Coronary Revascularization: A Report by the American College of Cardiology J. Am. Coll. Cardiol. 2009;53(6):530-553.

33. What did change was the rank order of physicians from highest to lowest cost. Typically, a given physician's ranking might move up or down one or two spots.

34. California's Health Insurance Exchange Builds Critical Outreach Network. *The California Report.* May 14, 2013. http://blogs.kqed.org/stateofhealth/2013/05/14/californias-health-insurance-exchange-builds-critical-outreach-network/

35. Births Methods of Delivery. Center for Disease Control 2010. http://www.cdc.gov/nchs/fastats/delivery.htm

36. The Kaiser Family Foundation. Kaiser Family Foundation Report on 2012 Employers Health Benefits Survey.2012. http://kff.org/report-section/ehbs-2012-section-1/. $15,745 for a family and $5615 for a single employee.

37. Baicker K, et al. The Oregon experiment—effects of Medicaid on clinical outcomes. N Engl J Med. 2013;368:1713-1722.

38. http://www.healthexchange.ca.gov/Pages/HBEXVisionMissionValues.aspx.

39. Covered California: Health Plans & Rates for 2014. http://coveredca.com/news/PDFs/CC_Health_Plans_Booklet.pdf

40. http://www.healthexchange.ca.gov/Pages/HBEXVisionMissionValues.aspx.

41. Issues for Manufacturer-Level Competitive Bidding for Durable Medical Equipment. GAO-11-337R, May 31, 2011 http://www.gao.gov/products/GAO-11-337R

42. Mitchell JB, Cromwell J. Medicaid mills: fact or fiction. Health Care Finance Rev. 1980 Summer;2(1):37-49.

43. Gawande A. The cost conundrum. *The New Yorker.* 2009;85(16):36-44

Index

Charge master, 45
Charges
  average charge, calculation, 114
  usage, 106
Cholelithiasis, 150
Chronic active hepatitis, blood-borne viral
  disease, 59–60
Chronic hepatitis, treatment, 64
Chronic kidney disease, anemia
  (consequence), 77
Chronic liver disease, 60
Chronic sinusitis
  ENT treatment, 104–105
  total charges, variation reduction graph,
    26f
  treatment cost, variation, 125
Clinical conversations, illumination, 154
Clinically warranted variation, existence, 20
Clinical outcomes, 6
CMS. *See* U.S. Centers for Medicare &
  Medicaid Services
Cochrane Collaboration, 57
Coefficient of variation, 138
Collaboration, importance, 91
Colonoscopy
  demand, increase, 63
  interval, examination, 159–160
  requirement, 104
  screening, 45
  suites, 161
  withdrawal time, 159
Co-morbid condition, impact, 25
Co-morbidity, control, 20
Computed tomography (CT) scan
  guidance, 65
  usage, 137
Content of care, improvement, 22
Control, attribution, 72
Cookbook medicine, 55
Cost, efficiency (contrast), 21
Cost reductions, opportunities, 13–14
Covered California, marketing, 165–167
Critical-care units (ventilator-associated
  pneumonia). incidence (decrease), 14

Current Procedural Terminology (CPT)
  codes, 115–116
  sorting, 116t
  usage, 87, 105–106

D

Dartmouth Atlas of Health Care, 7–8, 8f
  data, 11
Data
  analysis, benefits, 23
  anomaly, 5
  attribution, consistency, 107–109
  collection, initiating encounter, 28–29
  creation, 79
  filtering, 104–107
  gaps, 146–149
    search, 146–147
  gathering, 100–104, 116
    process, 78
  interaction, 149–151
  nonjudgmental approach, 76
  possession, 150
  presentation, observation, 92
  problem, 5, 21–22
    encounter, 146–149
    perception, 134
  production, 78
  robustness, 86–87
  unblinded data, presentation risk,
    121–122
  usage, 97
  warehouse, 103
    front end, variation-reduction team
      development, 77–78
Data sets, 160–161
  development, 91
  distribution, 133–134
  risk adjustment, 102
  search, 78
  variation, 139
Death panels, 5, 22
Degenerative osteoarthritis, ICD-9 codes, 87
Dermatology Department, variation-
  reduction team experience, 139
Diabetes, co-morbid condition, 20

Greenbranch Publishing

www.greenbranch.com (800) 933-3711